Holistic Menopause

A New Approach to Midlife Change

OTHER BOOKS BY JUDY HALL

Findhorn Press:
The Art of Psychic Protection
The Zodiac Pack
Hans Across Time

Other Publishers:
The Karmic Journey
Menopause Matters
The Astrology of a Prophet?
Principles of Past Life Therapy

Holistic Menopause

A New Approach to Midlife Change

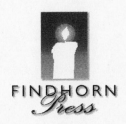

FINDHORN
Press

JUDY HALL

with
Dr Robert Jacobs MRCS LRCP

First published 1998

ISBN 1 899171 32 0

British Library Cataloguing-in-Publication Data.
A catalogue record for this book is available from the
British Library.

Cover design and book layout by David Gregson
Printed and bound WSOY, Finland

Published by
Findhorn Press
The Park, Findhorn, Forres IV36 0TZ, Scotland
tel +44 (0)1309 690582 • fax 690036
email thierry@findhorn.org
http://www.findhorn.org/findhornpress/

Contents

III: Body

IV: Mood

V: Mind

VI: Spirit

Appendix

List of Illustrations

Authors

Judy Hall and Dr Robert Jacobs are the authors of *Menopause Matters: A Practical Guide to the Menopause* (Element Books 1994). Dr Jacobs, a qualified medical doctor, has a private complementary medicine practice and combines Chinese medicine, Western herbalism, flower essences and vibratory medicine in his holistic approach to menopause. He has studied homoeopathy in Germany, and Chinese medicine in China.

Judy Hall, a highly experienced counsellor and writer, has a long-standing interest in complementary therapies including visualisation, emotional release work, journal-keeping and flower essences. She is the author of *The Zodiac Pack, Hands Across Time* and *The Art of Psychic Protection* (Findhorn Press) and *Principles of Past Life Therapy* (Thorsons).

Abbreviations

The following abbreviations are used throughout this book:

Alaskan	Alaskan Flower Essences
Bach	Bach Flower Remedies
Bloesem	Dutch Netherland Bloesem Essences
BMJ	British Medical Journal
Bush	Australian Bush Flower Essences
Cal	Californian Flower Essences
DA	Desert Alchemy
Findhorn	Findhorn Flower Essences
Him	Himalayan Flower Essences
HRT	Hormone Replacement Therapy
LE	Living Essences of Australian Flowers
Petaltone	Petaltone Essences
PMS	Premenstrual Syndrome
SA	South African Flower Essences
WDDTY	*What Doctors Don't Tell You* (magazine)

Foreword by Julie Felix

When I realised I would be 60 years old in 1998, I decided to give a celebration concert in London, and call it my 'Crone Concert'. I told friends of my intentions, and although they were enthusiastic about the concert, they said, "You mustn't call yourself a crone; it sounds so ugly. You look young for your age, so why tell people you will be 60?" They were being kind and I must admit I was pleased that they didn't think I looked like a 60-year-old! Nevertheless, I felt as though the wind had been taken out of my sails. Why did I have to pretend I was younger than I was? We all die, and unless we die young, we all grow old. Why is ageing considered a sin? Why are women so terrified of growing old? Shouldn't we celebrate having come this far along life's path rather than be ashamed of it? Our story is an unfolding one, and the more experiences we gather, the richer the narrative.

In our race to explain the wonders of nature in scientific terms, we have left behind some important keys that access our well-being as humans on this planet. Judy Hall has skilfully created a book that returns to us a most valuable key: the ability to honour and empower the 'Wise Woman', the 'Crone'. Judy reminds us of older cultures such as the Celts and the American Indians who honoured the grandmothers of the tribe. These older women were the teachers, the healers, the midwives. They not only assisted mothers in giving birth, but were also able to 'midwife the living through changes, endings, and dying'.

As women in today's society we face life's changes with fear and uncertainty. We are often the object of criticism and ridicule. Menopause is probably the hardest change of all. However, Judy tells us a different story — how menopause is a time for women to reclaim their true power. With courage she exposes the exploitation of menopausal women, especially by the medical profession and the pharmaceutical industry. "If menopause is to be reclaimed as a rite (or right) of passage rather than being accepted as a deficiency disease, then it is vital to take it back from the hands of the medical profession."

The author leads us by the hand through the dark forests of medical hype, sensational journalism and blatant lies; through the shadows of our deep feelings of inadequacy. Drawing on her background as an astrologer and counsellor Judy gives us spiritual and psychological insight into the situation every woman faces as she moves through the menopause years. Dr Robert Jacobs is a true knight serving the grail. He uses his knowledge of medicine to help women, not to exploit them. His traditional training as a doctor is augmented by his studies of Chinese medicine and other complementary practices. His work with vibrational medicine I find most appropriate since I personally believe this form of therapy will be essential as we move into the new millennium.

The combined knowledge of Judy and Rob makes this book a goldmine of information, especially in its comprehensive coverage of remedies such as flower essences. Moreover, it is designed in a way that allows the reader to participate in her own learning and healing process. Diary pages, question sheets and cycle charts are all provided to make this book a journey of self-discovery.

When I sing for teenagers, they are often surprised to discover that I am older than their parents. I have never taken HRT, and feel that my energy comes from my love of life. From my spirit. Sometimes, on a bad day, I start to doubt my beliefs. I feel depressed and I remember women who have told me that HRT counteracts depression. I think maybe this is the way I should go. Then I walk down to the fairy dell and listen to my 'inner voice'. I learn that I am sad; that sadness is part of the story, just as rain has its place amongst the seasons. Tears can be cleansing.

In one of my songs I write:

Virgin, girl child, madonna and old crone
The faces of the moon they let you know you're not alone

Judy Hall with this book lets us know we are not alone. We are all born; we all bleed; and eventually we all die. Menopause is the chance to make sense of it all. To pause and gather the gifts of life. To absorb the experiences, and to share our stories with those who are waiting to hear them. Thank you, Judy. Thank you for gathering your grandmother wisdom and for sharing it with us all. From one crone to another, *Gracias*!

JULIE FELIX
The Coromandel, New Zealand
January 1998

I: Change

Change is challenge to begin ever anew
A letting go, renouncing, moving on
To find an unpredicted life now shaped

Change

Early in 1991 I wrote a book called *The Wise Woman: A Natural Approach to the Menopause* with my partner Dr Robert Jacobs. This followed my own introduction to the disturbances which can signal the start of menopause, and the medical profession's answer to them. While I was writing it, there was little information around on menopause. For most women it was still viewed as something shameful and unmentionable. In the medical profession it had come to be regarded as a disease. Doctors were furiously prescribing HRT, but neither they nor the drug companies were giving women the full picture. Did doctors know it, I wonder? Do they know it now?

My co-writer, a doctor who had left conventional medicine, certainly had to dig deep into the medical literature to find relevant studies. At that stage he saw little to be concerned about except that there was a great deal of scientific knowledge about the processes of menopause and very little was being passed on to women. As a holistic doctor who combined many different approaches within his therapeutic work, he had much of the complementary medicine at his fingertips and knew how this could help women. Indeed, it was thanks to his guidance that I had found an answer to my own menopausal problems.

When writing that first book, we wanted to give an unbiased view so that women could make up their own minds about what treatment was appropriate for them, so we simply presented all the alternatives, with the evidence that was then available, and left it at that. I also wanted to bring menopause out of the closet, to show that it was a natural transition to another phase of life: a phase I called 'the wise woman'. I looked at the medical and social history of menopause, the fallacies and symptoms it engendered, the possibilities it created. I viewed it holistically, from the perspectives of body, mind, emotion and spirit. I spoke of menopause as a time when women could take possession of their own power.

The Wise Woman came out soon after Germaine Greer put menopause on the front page of almost every newspaper and into prime time television. Menopause became a major topic of conversation. But somehow women still didn't want to know. Yes, they wanted the facts about HRT and possible alternatives. But as to the mental, emotional and spiritual transition they were about to face, most of them would rather forget it. HRT was, of course, most helpful in this desire. They could go on bleeding. They could be symptomless, ageless. They could pretend nothing was happening.

By 1993, our publishers felt that the title I had chosen, *The Wise Woman,* was putting women off the book. They felt too that the section I had included on working with the Goddesses and ritual was 'too esoteric' for most women. We were aware that there was additional material we needed to incorporate — including new and somewhat disquieting evidence on HRT — and so we agreed to a rewrite. The publishers retitled the book *Menopause Matters: A Practical Approach to Midlife Change* and dropped much of the spiritual dimension. Sales soared. I did radio interviews and phone-ins, wrote articles, toured the country with menopause workshops, talked to many women, and then gradually returned to my 'other life' as a counsellor, astrologer and regression therapist. I still maintained my interest in menopause, however, and worked with women who happened, like me, to be in that phase of their life. Time passed. The book was overtaken by new ones which stressed the natural approach to menopause and emphasised that women should regain their power — but they said little about how to do this.

Then, one day in 1996, my co-author, who was still treating menopausal women, opened an alternative health magazine and read an article on Natural Menopause. Ninety per cent of it was his work, virtually word for word, with the source largely unacknowledged. He was relegated to a very small footnote at the end. At the time he was happy for the information to be more widely disseminated through any means. Clearly, though, his work had been ahead of its time, and now its time was coming.

More and more evidence was surfacing as to the fallacies being promoted about HRT, its safety and its preventive role in osteoporosis and heart disease. As one lone dissenting gynaecologist had said to me: "It's like using a sledgehammer to crack a nut." We felt certain that, whilst HRT may be beneficial for some women, there were many others who needed a different approach. We became aware of a need to communicate the possible dangers to women and to give constructive guidance on the alternative options open to them (holistic medicine is tailored to the person, not to a set of 'symptoms' assumed to be a disease). I had also begun to notice a need for a 'how to' book. Something had shifted. Suddenly women were contacting me, frantically trying to get hold of copies of *The Wise Woman* because they wanted to do the more spiritual inner work it contained. They needed a guidebook, something that would help them move through the confusing maze of conflicting advice and into the new phase of life that was being urged on them by so many writers on menopause. It seemed to be time to bring my attention back to the midlife transition. This book is the result.

— *Judy Hall*

Using This Book

This book is a guidebook. It is not intended to be a substitute for medical treatment and you are advised to consult a qualified practitioner before adopting any of the remedies suggested. It is designed to help you in two ways:

The first is to give you sufficient information to understand what is going on in your body and enable you to make informed choices about how to handle the changes that accompany the menopause. Menopause is not a disease. It is a life process. And as such it has several dimensions. So the book is divided into sections on the various aspects: Body, Mood, Mind and Spirit. Within each section you will find FactFiles that give you necessary information on specific topics. As some of the topics inevitably overlap between sections, you may find them in more than one place considered from varying perspectives. If you want to know what treatment is available for physical symptoms, or what the side-effects may be, for instance, you can easily look this up in Body. However, gentle medicine for the Mind, Mood and Spirit is also included in those specific sections.

The second purpose is to help you move through the transition and out the other side. Menopause is a time when many women feel uncertain, lost, unsure what comes next. New thoughts and feelings, urges and intuitions arise. The ToDo section of each topic is designed to help you explore what is happening in your body, your mind, your psyche and your life in general, and to find the way forward.

There is space in the book for 'Jottings', anything that occurs to you, new information, whatever you like. Nothing is more irritating than knowing you have seen something, or had an important insight, but not being able to remember exactly what or where. Don't be afraid to write in the book; it is a workbook and that is what it is intended for.

Buy yourself a notebook for the ToDo exercises (or start a computer file if you prefer). Choose a notebook that is attractive and special and use it to answer the questions or respond to the exercises, to write freely, and to record your thoughts and feelings. If you intend to return to the exercises at different times throughout the next year or so to see how your responses change, then you can leave sufficient space to do so. Be sure to date these entries clearly so that you can track what is happening. You can also incorporate an expanded menopause journal into this special book. You will find a 'menopause diary' helpful. A brief one is included in the pages that follow. This is intended to run over one month. It should be filled in every day if you are to gain the most from it. As you will see, it gathers together vital information and brings up insights not available in other ways. It has been incorporated into this book so that you will have all the information in one place, but if you wish to continue it you can photocopy the pages and keep them in a folder.

Some of the ToDo exercises will not relate to your own particular situation, in which case leave them out. But if exercises are relevant to you, then it is important to spend the time actually doing them, not just thinking about them. It will help you to both understand and integrate what is happening to you. The exercises in the Mood, Mind and Spirit sections of the book are designed to be ongoing, to lead you forward slowly. They are not to be rushed through in a few days. For this reason, you need to spread the book over several months. Indeed, it may take a year or two to work right through menopause and into the next phase of life. Most people will find it useful to read through the book first and then go back and work slowly through the relevant parts, dipping in and out of the different sections as appropriate.

▶ *ToDo*

▶ *Make a life statement*

Who are you? What do you want to say about yourself at this stage of your life? What is important to you?

Begin: I am a woman who . . .

(Return to this from time to time as you work through the book. Date each entry so that you can chart the changes in how you perceive yourself.)

What do you wish for yourself?

We shall come back to this statement later.

The Menopause: A Medical History

In tribal societies menopause has always been seen as a rite of passage. Women were given the space and care they needed. Herbs and rituals were available to them. When they had passed through menopause, they were honoured as wise women, grandmother elders. Even in non-tribal societies, until the rise of a monied and leisured class of women in the nineteenth century, women who survived to menopause were treated by herbalists and wise women. It was a normal part of life. In the nineteenth century, however, first physicians and then surgeons took over. This was not a result of an altruistic surge of interest in women's well-being. These men were self-created 'experts' offering a service for which they engineered a demand and expected high remuneration. In both Europe and America they found a reservoir of willing victims. Nineteenth-century women, on the whole, looked up to men as their natural masters.

Suddenly menopause became a disease with symptoms that apparently required invasive and toxic treatment. The eminent English Victorian gynaecologist Edward Tilt, who viewed menopausal women as hysterical and morbid, with criminal leanings, advocated sedatives, morphine, syrup of iron and potassium, bandaging of the limbs and restraint with abdominal belts, supplemented above all by bleeding. According to Dr Tilt, menopausal headaches were caused by an excess of blood in the head. So he applied leeches to the nape of the neck and behind the ears.

Tilt would later be referred to as a 'bleeder, puker and purger'. However, Dr Andrew Currier, who made this comment, and his colleagues were not much better. Currier still used leeches and advocated total removal of the uterus and ovaries. Naturally this caused even more symptoms, which he put down to vicious habits, use of substances such as alcohol, chloral or opium, or, worse still, excessive sexual indulgence. In his unforgiving view, menopause was a socio-economic phenomenon, the result of such unwomanly occupations as metal-working, labouring, cooking and laundering, not to mention selling fish. Such women were 'pitiful spectacles of decrepit and wrinkled and worn out creatures'.

Nor did the psychoanalysts treat menopause with much compassion. Freud, whose patients tended to be middle-aged, middle-class women, viewed menopause as a time of potential crisis and hysteria when even previously placid women could become quarrelsome and obstinate. One of his followers, Helene Deutsch, promulgated the theory that women were only of service to the species as long as they were producing children. After that, their useful life was finished — a view which still has its adherents today. Jung was gentler with women. He saw midlife as the time when the previously unlived life would take over and demand to be expressed. So women who had up until then been meek, mild, home-loving and obedient to their husband would suddenly become much more dominant and outgoing. They would begin to make a life outside the home, to put their talents to work. If they ignored this urge, then they would exhibit psychosomatic symptoms or retreat into 'nervous breakdown'.

Menopause remained within the domain of the surgeons, however, especially in the United States, until the development of oestrogen therapy, or HRT, over thirty years ago. The first oestrogen came from the urine of pregnant horses (some of it still does). Hundreds of women died of breast and uterine cancer before someone decided to add progestogen to the mix. By the 1970s in the States and the 80s in the UK, HRT was being heralded as the woman's cure-all. "It keeps women out of the orthopaedic wards, the divorce courts and the madhouse," said one eminent consultant gynaecologist at a London hospital. Books, and doctors, touted HRT as the panacea for all women's ills, physical or psychological. Menopause became big business, in the pharmaceutical industry at least. Business worth millions of pounds a year.

The Menopause Machine

The menopause machine grinds inexorably on. Its fuel is a collective desire for youth at all costs. Its tools are propaganda, fear and the aura of power attached to the medical profession. It has generated a fear of old age never before known, which has a powerful hold on women. A hold that can only be broken by informed choice.

Today, the leaflets on menopause that you pick up in your doctor's surgery are likely to be disguised advertising for HRT, as they have mostly been produced by the drug companies or drug-company-funded organisations. (Look carefully at the small print or at the end-of-year reports of these bodies if you have access to them: even organisations claiming to be independent are often dependent for funding on donations from the pharmaceutical industries.) The menopause groups now being held at surgeries are usually funded by the drug companies for the same covert, profit-orientated reason. If a demand for HRT is created through 'women's awareness', the pharmaceutical industry will be only too pleased to supply it. When I gave talks on natural medicine at a doctor's surgery, I was asked by the practice nurse not to mention the side-effects of HRT or the increasing evidence of its dangers because it would mean losing the funding from a drug company. Vested interests make the passing on of unbiased, objective information impossible.

What is Menopause?

Most emphatically, menopause is not a disease. It is a rite of passage on a par with birth, puberty, sexual initiation and death. Strictly speaking, menopause is the last menstrual period you have. (It can be translated as 'the moon of pause'.) But the word has come to encompass the whole period of hormonal change leading up to this climactic event, and the time immediately following it.

Menopause is a natural process of midlife change and transition. It has definite physical indications — menstrual periods stop, for instance — but it is much more than this. It is something that happens on emotional, mental and spiritual levels as well. There is an imperative behind menopause: change, become more aware, live your unlived life to the full, move into what you may be. Whilst there are aspects of menopause that apply to every woman, you will experience menopause in your own unique, individual way. As it is part of your overall life experience, all that you are and have already gone through in your life will contribute to your menopausal years. And to what comes after.

Each of us has a body clock which sets out the cycles and seasons of our life and has certain trigger points built into it. These trigger points are programmed for roughly the same age in everyone but there may be a leeway of five or even ten years in individual women. Puberty, for instance, signals the hormonal influx that accompanies adolescence. But it may happen to girls as young as nine or ten and equally may not occur until fifteen, sixteen or even seventeen.

At a certain point in midlife, the body clock will trigger the hormonal changes that lead to cessation of ovulation and, consequently, the end of menstruation. This is how it is meant to be. Your body is designed like this. Menopause is not a deficiency. It is not that the body 'runs out of eggs' but rather that nature has decided that it is time to move on to something else. The Chinese believe that vital life force is lost through menstrual bleeding, and so menopause is a way of stopping this loss, and is therefore life-enhancing.

The fluctuating levels of hormones which accompany this bodily change are responsible for many of the physical and mood disturbances that may accompany menopause as your body tries to adapt (disturbances which I have called symptoms without intending to imply that they are symptomatic of disease). The body is a resilient organism and, left to itself, it will usually make the change quite smoothly. The psyche sometimes takes a little time to adjust. Not much has been heard about the soul this century, but it is now rallying women to its call. Occasionally a few gremlins get into the works (quite often these gremlins are factors that you yourself contribute: food, stress, resistance, crisis) and you may need a little help.

▶ *To Do:*

What does menopause mean to you?

Choose a time when you will not be disturbed and sit quietly for a few moments. Then, when you are ready, write down everything the menopause means to you. Do not censor. Don't worry where these thoughts and feelings come from. Just let it all flow onto the paper:

What was menopause like for your mother and other female members of the family?

Did you know what was going on?

What were you told about menopause by family and friends?

The beliefs that you inherit through your mother, the experience she had, the way she dealt with her own menopause, the messages she gave you, the deep dark secrets she kept, all have a bearing on your own menopausal passage. We shall return to these later in the book but, for the time being, mull over what you have just written and if anything further comes to mind, add it to what you have already written.

The Physiology of Menopause

Before menopause, the ovaries produce female sex hormones: mainly oestrogens and progesterone. As menopause gets under way, the level of oestrogen in the body drops. This causes the pituitary gland at the base of the brain to secrete raised levels of gonadotrophins (hormones which stimulate the release of sex hormones by the ovaries) in an attempt to increase oestrogen production and keep menstruation going. This attempt ultimately fails but it is the reason for the fluctuating levels of oestrogen found in menopausal women, which in turn trigger many of the more unpleasant side-effects: hot flushes, night sweats, a dry vagina and other physical conditions. As hormones are the chemical messengers of the body, the physiology of menopause can also have a profound effect on mood and mental competence.

At the same time, or much earlier in some women, progesterone production falls. Progesterone is produced towards the end of the menstrual cycle. If ovulation (the release of an egg from the ovary) has not occurred for any reason, and there are several, then progesterone will not be produced but the lining of the womb will still be shed (a period) as it will not be required for pregnancy. So there is little outward sign that progesterone production has virtually ceased. Oestrogen production may go on for years until the body's clock signals it is time for a change.

Oestrogen and progesterone usually hold each other in check, but without one or the other the function is exaggerated. Even when progesterone is still being produced up to menopause, the two hormones get out of balance and the body chemistry goes awry. As body chemistry is linked to many physiological processes, this imbalance affects not only the physical level but also mood and mental functioning and competence. Eventually the body begins to make oestrogen through the adrenal glands and the body's fat stores and oestrogen levels can be as high as 40% of pre-menopausal levels. Progesterone production, however, does not recommence.

If a woman has been making less progesterone for some time, perhaps for as long as ten or more years before menopause begins, then the two hormones may become seriously out of balance, leading to oestrogen dominance. This dominance is increasing in the industrial world because of certain pollutants that act as false oestrogens and mimic oestrogen function in the body. Such pollutants are found in water and in food (a good reason for choosing organic food wherever possible). The symptoms of oestrogen dominance[1] mimic PMS and menopausal indications, which may be why some 'menopauses' seem to go on for ever.

▶ *FactFile*

Menopause is the result of decreasing production by the body of the female sex hormones, oestrogen and progesterone. As these hormones regulate the menstrual cycle and its associated fertility, menopause signals the end of menstruation and the cessation of reproductive capacity.

The average age for menopause has been 51 for as long as records have been kept. It can occur in the early 40s and may go on until the late 50s.

By age 54 80% of women are one year past menopause.

In the 17th century, only 28% of women reached menopause. Now 95% of women in the developed world do so because of increased life expectancy.

The human female is the only mammal to experience menopause.

The only certain test for menopause is to measure gonadotrophin levels. If the ratio of FSH to LH (follicle-stimulating hormone to luteinising hormone) is greater than three to one, then ovarian function has ceased and you are definitely post-menopausal. Blood tests by a doctor, or saliva tests by a complementary practitioner, will establish hormone levels.

Menopause Indications

Menopause is not an illness or a deficiency. It is a naturally occurring process of midlife change which may be accompanied by physical, mental and emotional indications often called symptoms.

▶ *FactFile*

20% of women have no menopausal indications other than cessation of menstrual periods.

10% of women have severe and debilitating disturbances ('symptoms') which may need treatment.

Most women experience slight physical disturbances as hormone levels adjust themselves. Left alone, these disturbances will usually soon disappear but they can be helped with complementary therapies.

Many women experience emotional disturbances around the time of menopause as they adjust to their new role in life.

Mental disturbances, such as forgetfulness and 'woolly-headed-ness' are common. Simple remedies can help.

Medically recognised menopausal indications: hot flushes, sweats, dizziness, insomnia, osteoporosis, apprehension, cardiovascular changes, palpitations, headaches, anxiety, urge incontinence, libido changes, menstrual changes, arthropathies (painful joints), loss of concentration, depression, skin atrophy (thinning), formication (crawling sensation of the skin), globus hystericus (lump in the throat).

No one will experience all of these indications. Most women have two or three at most and then only for a short time.

Most common indication: Hot flushes or sweats are experienced by 75% of women.

A hot flush is the only 'symptom' unique to menopause.

Hot flush: Felt as a 'rush of heat' in various parts of the body which may be accompanied by reddening of the skin. A hot flush is a physiologically measurable event. Skin temperature rises as blood vessels dilate and heartbeat increases.

Average duration: 3 minutes but can last between 0.5 and 60 minutes.

Rate of occurrence: 1 to 100 times per week

Some of the supposedly rare disturbances, such as a lump in the throat or a feeling of crawling and itching on the skin, are not always recognised by the medical profession. Nor are they immediately obvious to sufferers as pertaining to midlife change. However, many women report these rather bizarre sensations.

▶ *HotTips*

▶ *Coping with hot flushes and night sweats*

Wear loose, light layers of natural fibres. Avoid tight neck- and waistbands.

At night, lie on bath towels or sleep in a cotton towelling robe — it's easier than changing the whole bed. Use cotton sheets where possible.

Stick your feet out from under the duvet to cool yourself down quickly.

Sleep alone.

Switch to Earl Grey tea (bergamot oil helps).

Spray yourself with Evian water in which you have soaked thyme leaves.

Put your feet in a bowl of hot water.

Learn to recognise, and avoid, triggers such as coffee.

Keep the Bush Flower essence *Mulla Mulla* handy and take a few drops when necessary.

Hot flushes can be enjoyable. Learn to go with the surge of powerful warmth.

▶ *Jottings*

Am I Menopausal...?

Ask most people (especially men) to describe a typical menopausal woman and they will portray someone red, hot, perspiring, probably overweight, and most certainly irrational and prone to odd behaviour. Ask the age and it will probably be 'in the mid-50s'. This is the stereotyped picture that Western society has evolved of a rather peculiar and pitiful creature. It is, however, far from true.

Little wonder then that few woman actually recognise themselves as approaching 'The Change' unless they fit this stereotype. They may put little idiosyncrasies down to 'my age', but how many women in their 40s acknowledge the subtle onset of pre-menopausal changes. Even when they get into the 50s, they tend to be reluctant to admit, even to themselves, that they have become menopausal. It is still something to be ashamed of, something to hide. The onset of old age. Later we shall see just how fallacious this view is. But in the meantime it may help to identify the many and varied ways that midlife change can affect you. The changes occur not only in your physical body, but also on an emotional, mental and spiritual level.

▶ *To Do*

Describe how you picture a menopausal woman. Include the kind of symptoms you expect to have:

▶ *Menopause*

Tick the boxes which apply to you:

Menstrual periods stopped ☐

Menstrual periods erratic, scanty, heavy ☐

Hot flushes ☐

Night sweats ☐

Dry vagina ☐

Mood swings ☐

Loss of libido ☐

Aged between 42 and 58 ☐

If you have ticked several boxes, it is likely that you are entering, in the process of or leaving menopause. A hormone test can tell you for sure.

There is, however, a much broader range of 'symptoms' that may affect you:

Tick the boxes that apply to you:

Hot flushes ☐

Palpitations ☐

Night sweats ☐

Cystitis ☐

Excessively hot or cold feet ☐

Incontinence ☐

Irregular periods ☐

Aphasia (word loss) ☐

Scanty or heavy menstrual bleeding ☐

Osteoporosis ☐

Ageing and weakness of the skin ☐

Decrease in height ☐

Vaginal dryness or discharge ☐

Low calcium levels ☐

Flooding ☐

Mood swings ☐

Increased PMS ☐

Depression ☐

Mastitis ☐

Indecisiveness ☐

Headaches ☐

Feelings of inadequacy ☐

Insomnia ☐

Irritability ☐

Memory loss ☐

Vivid dreams ☐

Tiredness and lethargy ☐

Anxiety ☐

Weight gain ☐

Agitation ☐

Aching bones, muscles or limbs ☐

Extreme elation ☐

Bloatedness ☐

Tearfulness ☐

Flatulence ☐

Change in libido ☐

Digestive problems ☐

Fearfulness ☐

Occasional dizzy spells ☐

Confusion ☐

Tingling or crawling of skin ☐

Agoraphobia or other phobias ☐

Gum disease and halitosis ☐

Irrational feelings ☐

Food allergies ☐

Loss of purpose ☐

Spots ☐

Loss of concentration ☐

Hair loss ☐

Mental blanks ☐

Whilst very few of the above indications are specifically meno-pausal, all or any of them can affect you at midlife. If you have ticked more than three or four, then you are likely to be undergoing pre-menopausal hormone changes or the actual menopause itself, or you are experiencing the accelerated change of a 'midlife crisis'. Working through this book will help you to sort out which is which, and how they intertwine. Either way, there are many constructive paths open to you now which will enable you to take charge of your life and health.

▶ ### *Oestrogen dominance*

Water retention and swelling ☐

Breast tenderness and fibrocystic disease ☐

PMS ☐

Mood swings ☐

Depression ☐

Loss of libido ☐

Heavy or irregular periods ☐

History of amenorrhoea (no periods) ☐

Fibroids ☐

Craving for sweets ☐

Weight gain with fat deposited at thighs and hips ☐

Taking HRT ☐

Hysterectomy but ovaries remain ☐

The above may indicate oestrogen dominance[1] and lack of progesterone rather than menopause itself. It is worth having your hormone levels properly tested. (You may need additional progesterone — see page 91 — or natural remedies to promote hormonal balance).

...Or Am I Having a Midlife Crisis?

(Tick the boxes that apply to you)

Have you lost your sense of identity? ☐

Are you tense, anxious, confused? ☐

Do you feel your life is out of control? ☐

Are you facing a period of turbulence? ☐

Has your partner left? ☐

Do you suspect your husband is having an affair? ☐

Are you having, or contemplating, an affair? ☐

Has a child recently left home or is about to? ☐

Do you have a young child to cope with? ☐

Have you or your partner been made redundant? ☐

Do you have financial worries? ☐

Do you fear getting old? ☐

Do you feel your sexual attractiveness is waning? ☐

Do you feel the best part of your life is over? ☐

Are you suffering from unexplained depression? ☐

Do you feel your life is going in the wrong direction? ☐

Do you feel you are stuck in a dead end job? ☐

Do you desperately want to make a change? ☐

Tick more than one or two and you may well be having a midlife crisis. Of course it is possible to be menopausal *and* have a midlife crisis. But don't worry, this is an opportunity to sort things out and the menopause is usually followed by a period of zest and renewed interest in life.

Medically Induced Menopause

As mentioned earlier, for many years hysterectomy was seen as a 'cure' for menopausal disturbances, especially for symptoms such as heavy bleeding, although any symptom at all was used as an excuse. If your child-bearing days were over, the surgeons said, then you did not need your womb. The role of the ovaries in hormone production was not understood, so all the reproductive organs were removed. Consequently thousands of women were precipitated even deeper into menopause. Even for non-menopausal women who were still menstruating, surgeons found many 'reasons' to perform hysterectomy.

Hysterectomy is still carried out today for a variety of gynaecological conditions. If you have a hysterectomy that includes the removal of your ovaries, then you have an immediate menopause. If, however, you have a hysterectomy that leaves your ovaries in place, you will experience menopause at the age at which you would naturally have done so had you not had the hysterectomy (which may be many years later). The only difference is that you will not have menstrual periods in the meantime. As surgeons often do not mention that menopause will occur in normal timing after womb-only hysterectomy, its onset can be quite a shock, especially if the hysterectomy has been performed several years previously. If this happens to you, you will still need to address the other dimensions of midlife change on the feeling, mental and spiritual levels so that you can move into a different phase of life.

Nowadays most surgeons prescribe HRT in the form of oestrogen only to help you over the initial post-operative period and many take the view that women who undergo hysterectomy, no matter what their age, should stay on HRT indefinitely to prevent future osteoporosis. As there are now serious doubts being raised about the role of oestrogen in preventing osteoporosis, and because of the risk of oestrogen becoming dominant in your body, if you have been given this advice it would probably be sensible to look into the claims being made for natural progesterone (see pages 91 and 115) under the guidance of an appropriately qualified practitioner.

The other medically induced menopause comes about when Tamoxifen is prescribed for breast cancer patients. This causes an artificial cessation of menstruation and leads to menopause. Again, in addition to the issues that one has to face in coping with breast cancer, there will be menopausal disturbances on all levels to deal with. Natural medicine can be of great help here, as can appropriate counselling (which is offered at some hospitals but not others). If you feel you need additional help, don't be afraid to ask your doctor to refer you to an appropriately trained counsellor.

It has been suggested that natural progesterone can protect against any risk involved in the use of Tamoxifen (see FactFile), as it appears to have a protective function against cancer.[2] (The cream should be applied externally to the skin, but not to the breasts, under the supervision of a qualified practitioner who can monitor the results.)

▶ *FactFile*

There are an increasing number of questions about the safety of Tamoxifen (a weak oestrogen) and the advisability of its use. A possible link between Tamoxifen and endometrial cancer has been found.[3]

There are alternatives to hysterectomy. Laser surgery can remove the lining of the uterus but the procedure carries its own dangers. Reconstructive surgery may be possible. Check out the alternatives. Herbs can help. If necessary, seek a second opinion before agreeing to surgery.[4]

▶ *Jottings:*

References

1   *Natural Progesterone*, John Lee MD. BLL Publishing, California, 1993

2   The Natural Progesterone Information Service leaflet: *Some Basic Information on Natural Progesterone* (see Resources section)

3   *What Doctors Don't Tell You*, Lynne McTaggart. Thorsons, London, 1996 (*WDDTY* Vol. 5 Nos. 2, 3, 4)

4   *No More Hysterectomies*, Dr Vicky Hufnagel. Thorsons, London, 1990 (*WDDTY* Vol.7 No.1)

Reclaiming Power

Menopause is the time when you can reclaim your true power as a woman. It is also a time when you can reclaim your body. Indeed, if menopause is to be reinstated as a rite (or right) of passage rather than being accepted as a deficiency disease, then it is vital to take it back from the hands of the medical profession. You submit to the 'power over' aspect of medicine whenever you unquestioningly allow a doctor to tell you what you need or what you are 'suffering' from. You hand your power over whenever a doctor writes a prescription without telling you exactly what is in it and what it will do. You lose your power whenever a gynaecologist takes away a part of your body without your informed consent. You have no power if you unquestioningly accept as the best option that which you are told is 'good for you'. In these circumstances, the 'cure' comes from outside. It is not based on your power to take control of your own bodily processes or to make decisions about your own life.

A study conducted among cancer patients in the USA showed that those who assertively questioned their doctor's decisions had a better prognosis than those who passively accepted what was told to them and meekly went along with their doctor's conclusions. As menopause is not a disease, it is even more important to question medical assumptions.

As we have seen, for almost a century hysterectomy was routinely prescribed to 'cure' menopause. Over the last thirty years or so, HRT has taken over. Whilst menopause remains in the hands of the pharmaceutical industry, all efforts to relieve its symptoms are driven purely by the quest for profit, not by concern for women's well-being. Medical menopause masks a lack of wholeness and balance, a condition for which healing can only come from inside. If you listen to your body, and your intuition, it can tell you what you need. When you have true knowing, rather than the half-truths and fallacies that pass for information, you are empowered as a woman. Only then can you find a way through midlife transition that is exactly right for you. This book seeks to guide you. It is not infallible but it may help you to find the answers.

II: Diary

*Change is being lost in strange unrealness
to end or begin*

Keeping a Menopause Diary

The simplest way to keep track of what is happening to you during midlife change is a daily diary. You will find one set out in the pages that follow. The diary should be filled in at least once a day for three months but you may like to jot down important events as they occur, especially when keeping track of 'symptoms' and passing moods. A brief note in the pages which follow is all that is required, but keeping a longer, more comprehensive menopause journal offers an opportunity to express your feelings more fully. This can be combined with the exercises throughout this book. You may like to create a special time for yourself, just before you go to bed perhaps, when you can recall and report on your day. Many women find that honouring what is going in their bodies and their intimate thoughts is healing, supportive and life-enhancing.

The diary will give you useful data at a glance. No more wondering exactly when you last had a period, for example — the pattern and any irregularities will immediately be apparent. Moreover, shading in the section for 'bleeding' means that you can instantly spot prolonged or heavy bleeding. It will also give you much more subtle information, enabling you to link apparently disparate events such as, for instance, the food you eat with the hot flushes you experience. It shows you which treatments are effective, and may indicate which ones are causing unwanted side-effects. It also aids in linking stress-creating situations with the symptoms they produce.

Diary

Date:

Day of cycle:

Bleeding:

Moon phase:

Mood:

Indications:

Events:

Sleep:

Dreams:

Food:

Treatments:

Diary

Date:

Day of cycle:

Bleeding:

Moon phase:

Mood:

Indications:

Events:

Sleep:

Dreams:

Food:

Treatments:

Diary

Date:

Day of cycle:

Bleeding:

Moon phase:

Mood:

Indications:

Events:

Sleep:

Dreams:

Food:

Treatments:

Diary

Date:

Day of cycle:

Bleeding:

Moon phase:

Mood:

Indications:

Events:

Sleep:

Dreams:

Food:

Treatments:

Diary

Date:

Day of cycle:

Bleeding:

Moon phase:

Mood:

Indications:

Events:

Sleep:

Dreams:

Food:

Treatments:

Diary

Date:

Day of cycle:

Bleeding:

Moon phase:

Mood:

Indications:

Events:

Sleep:

Dreams:

Food:

Treatments:

Diary

Date:

Day of cycle:

Bleeding:

Moon phase:

Mood:

Indications:

Events:

Sleep:

Dreams:

Food:

Treatments:

Diary

Date:

Day of cycle:

Bleeding:

Moon phase:

Mood:

Indications:

Events:

Sleep:

Dreams:

Food:

Treatments:

Diary

Date:

Day of cycle:

Bleeding:

Moon phase:

Mood:

Indications:

Events:

Sleep:

Dreams:

Food:

Treatments:

Diary

Date:

Day of cycle:

Bleeding:

Moon phase:

Mood:

Indications:

Events:

Sleep:

Dreams:

Food:

Treatments:

Diary

Date:

Day of cycle:

Bleeding:

Moon phase:

Mood:

Indications:

Events:

Sleep:

Dreams:

Food:

Treatments:

Diary

Date:

Day of cycle:

Bleeding:

Moon phase:

Mood:

Indications:

Events:

Sleep:

Dreams:

Food:

Treatments:

Diary

Date:

Day of cycle:

Bleeding:

Moon phase:

Mood:

Indications:

Events:

Sleep:

Dreams:

Food:

Treatments:

Diary

Date:

Day of cycle:

Bleeding:

Moon phase:

Mood:

Indications:

Events:

Sleep:

Dreams:

Food:

Treatments:

Diary

Date:

Day of cycle:

Bleeding:

Moon phase:

Mood:

Indications:

Events:

Sleep:

Dreams:

Food:

Treatments:

Diary

Date:

Day of cycle:

Bleeding:

Moon phase:

Mood:

Indications:

Events:

Sleep:

Dreams:

Food:

Treatments:

Diary

Date:

Day of cycle:

Bleeding:

Moon phase:

Mood:

Indications:

Events:

Sleep:

Dreams:

Food:

Treatments:

Diary

Date:

Day of cycle:

Bleeding:

Moon phase:

Mood:

Indications:

Events:

Sleep:

Dreams:

Food:

Treatments:

Diary

Date:

Day of cycle:

Bleeding:

Moon phase:

Mood:

Indications:

Events:

Sleep:

Dreams:

Food:

Treatments:

Diary

Date:

Day of cycle:

Bleeding:

Moon phase:

Mood:

Indications:

Events:

Sleep:

Dreams:

Food:

Treatments:

Date:

Day of cycle:

Bleeding:

Moon phase:

Mood:

Indications:

Events:

Sleep:

Dreams:

Food:

Treatments:

Diary

Date:

Day of cycle:

Bleeding:

Moon phase:

Mood:

Indications:

Events:

Sleep:

Dreams:

Food:

Treatments:

Diary

Date:

Day of cycle:

Bleeding:

Moon phase:

Mood:

Indications:

Events:

Sleep:

Dreams:

Food:

Treatments:

Diary

Date:

Day of cycle:

Bleeding:

Moon phase:

Mood:

Indications:

Events:

Sleep:

Dreams:

Food:

Treatments:

Diary

Date:

Day of cycle:

Bleeding:

Moon phase:

Mood:

Indications:

Events:

Sleep:

Dreams:

Food:

Treatments:

Diary

Date:

Day of cycle:

Bleeding:

Moon phase:

Mood:

Indications:

Events:

Sleep:

Dreams:

Food:

Treatments:

Diary

Date:

Day of cycle:

Bleeding:

Moon phase:

Mood:

Indications:

Events:

Sleep:

Dreams:

Food:

Treatments:

Date:

Day of cycle:

Bleeding:

Moon phase:

Mood:

Indications:

Events:

Sleep:

Dreams:

Food:

Treatments:

Diary

Date:

Day of cycle:

Bleeding:

Moon phase:

Mood:

Indications:

Events:

Sleep:

Dreams:

Food:

Treatments:

Diary

Date:

Day of cycle:

Bleeding:

Moon phase:

Mood:

Indications:

Events:

Sleep:

Dreams:

Food:

Treatments:

Diary Entries

Date

Always date your entry with the month and day. This enables you to track events quickly, especially if you are also keeping a detailed journal. If you do need to seek medical advice, then you have an instant record of what occurred and when — which is useful, as menopause is a time when you may less easily recall detail.

Day of cycle

Entering your cycle day will enable you to see the variation in the pattern of your periods and link it to fluctuations of mood and physical symptoms such as increased PMS, backache or headaches. It enables you to pinpoint where in your cycle your libido is at its strongest, and to fit your lovemaking to the rise and fall of desire. If you are taking HRT, natural progesterone or other treatments that need to be tied to the menstrual cycle, the correct day can quickly be identified.

Early in menopause, the duration of the cycle may lengthen or shorten and may well swing between extremes. After menstruation ceases, many women report still being aware of exactly where in their monthly cycle they would be if they were still bleeding. If you have had a menopause surgically induced by hysterectomy which left your ovaries intact, then you will still be going through the ovulation cycle. This cycle will regulate your inner experience and may well affect your outer world too.

Bleeding

If you use a red pen to shade in days of bleeding, filling one-third of the box for light bleeding, two thirds for normal and a full box for heavy, you will quickly identify prolonged or 'abnormal' bleeding (for which medical advice should always be sought) and days of 'spotting' which may be linked to treatments being taken. Prolonged or frequent bleeding, which may well cause tiredness or anaemia, may need appropriate action (many of the complementary therapies regulate bleeding).

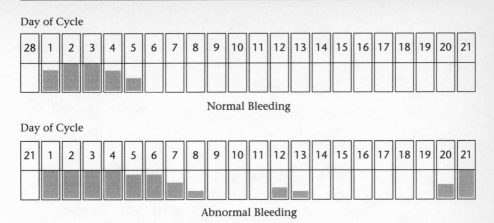

Day of Cycle

28	1	2	3	4	5	6	7	8	9	10	11	12	13	14	15	16	17	18	19	20	21

Normal Bleeding

Day of Cycle

21	1	2	3	4	5	6	7	8	9	10	11	12	13	14	15	16	17	18	19	20	21

Abnormal Bleeding

Fig 1: Normal and abnormal patterns of bleeding

Moon phase

Many years ago the moon regulated women's lives. At the dark of the moon they gathered in the menstrual hut to dream their dreams and regain their strength. It was a time of introspection, processing and renewal. Then, as the moon waxed again, they would return to the world refreshed and ready to put their visions into action.

You can still use this ancient cycle to enrich your life. The dark of the moon is a time for introspection, for moving into one's depths, dreaming the dream, processing all that has happened over the preceding weeks. The new moon is the time to come out into the world again, to begin new projects, to bring that inner vision out to the light. The full moon is a creative time when you can take action and make your visions manifest. The last quarter moon brings things to fruition. Then, as the moon withdraws to dark again, you can begin the movement inward once more.

If you are menstruating, you may find that the cycle changes as menopause draws near and the fertility cycle winds its way to a close. If you are no longer menstruating and have lost touch with your own cycle, the moon cycle can guide your inner life, the ebb and flow of withdrawal and action. Either way, taking counsel from the moon and withdrawing from the world at the dark of the moon brings an inner peace that can then be taken out into daily life.

Mood

Mood fluctuations at and around menopause can be violent and extreme, seemingly without reason or rationale. Panic attacks may strike without warning. Tears may be followed by elation, anger by ravenous hunger. Many women put it down to 'my age' or 'my hormones'. But there may well be a hidden reason, one related to food, blood sugar levels, menstrual cycle or the events in our lives. A chocolate binge may stuff down depressed or angry thoughts, but it may also indicate an underlying blood sugar disturbance that would be much better dealt with by a slow-release carbohydrate diet. A daily diary is the best way to identify such links.

In the abbreviated diary in this book, there is room for short entries to be jotted down during the day. But if you are keeping a longer journal, then you will have more room to explore in full the feelings and emotions that strike you 'out of the blue'. Take the time to write everything down without censoring it, no matter how trivial or 'wrong' it may feel. Somewhere you will find the clue you need. It may all feel like doom and gloom, but trying to make positive entries as well will help you to see what is working. This approach also pays dividends in an increased sense of well-being as it focuses attention away from the drain of pessimistic and negative thoughts.

Indications

This is the place for all the 'symptoms' you are encountering. If you are having frequent and prolonged hot flushes, note down the time and duration. Note the less obvious signs, such as aching joints, loss of memory or dry skin, and then compare this box with the food box for the day and a day or two preceding it. You will quickly spot whether coffee or hot and spicy food is contributing to your hot flushes. The occasional loss of a word can be a sign of hormonal imbalance, but it can also relate to food allergy (the most common types involving dairy or wheat products). This section will also enable you to monitor the efficacy of treatments and to establish what is working and what can be discarded.

Events

Jot down the events in your life (and if necessary explore them in your expanded journal). This can be an important clue as to how your menopausal 'symptoms' are a response to your lifestyle. The effect of stress is well known, and the extra adrenaline overload may throw your body even further out of balance. And remember, stress does not just arise from the difficult times — even joyful events can affect your body.

Sleep

Insomnia and disturbed sleep are common occurrences at menopause. Inability to fall asleep despite being tired, falling asleep only to jerk awake in the middle of the night, or waking early in the morning may all happen. This may be linked to the menstrual cycle, vivid dreams being common in the days leading up to a period, for instance. But it could equally be linked to stress or to symptoms such as night sweats. In Chinese medicine, waking at a certain time is an indication of energetic disturbance of a particular organ, so it can be a useful diagnostic tool.

Herbal sleeping preparations and self-hypnosis tapes are most effective in combating insomnia but a good first step may be to deal with the stress in your life and learn to relax. A milky drink or something to eat at bedtime is often recommended for people who have trouble falling asleep, but camomile tea induces sleep within twenty minutes in at least 60% of people and is well worth trying.

Dreams

Vivid and sometimes terrifying dreams are common around menopause, especially at the time when you are, or would be, menstruating. Keeping a note in this diary and then further amplifying the dream in your extended journal will help you to work with these messages from your subconscious mind. You may also find that certain foods trigger dreams. Cheese has long been associated with nightmares, for instance. You may also find a link between night sweats and vivid dreams or between the events of your day and this nocturnal processing.

Date: Feb	1	2	3	4	5	6	7
Day of Cycle	18	19	20	21	22	1	2
Bleeding						▓	▓
Moon	○						◗
Mood	Depressed weepy Can't cope at work	I am a failure	Don't feel like sex	BAD!!	Irritable Worried about Ann		Depressed Can't concentrate
Indications	Hot flush Hot flush	Night sweats Hot flush	Dragging ache Tender breasts	Hot flush Hot flush pm.	Headache Night sweats	Hot sweats Nausea	Tired Dizzy Feeling faint
Events	Important meeting goes badly No time to shop	Weekly shop and washing Leave Ironing	Jim insists on sex	Flowers from Jim Ann phones unhappy and homesick	Row with Jim – wouldn't go out with him	Leave work early	Stayed off work Row with Jim
Sleep	Poor	Poor	Awake 'til 2		None	Little	None
Dreams	'Falling'	Can't remember			Horrible nightmare	Vivid	
Food	Coffee Business lunch Wine, coffee coffee	Six chocolate bars		Liquid lunch Coffeepot full			Box of chocolates Ready-meal
Treatment	Paracetamol		Aspirin		4 doses of Paracetamol		

Fig 2: Sample diary pages

8	9	10	11	12	13	14	15
3	4	5	6	7	8	9	10
					☾	●	☽
Can't cope	Depressed	Weepy Feel under pressure	Miserable	am: Why bother pm: Feeling good	Hopeful – feel very different today		Optimistic
Tired Dizzy	Exhausted Can't wake up all day	Hot flushes Can't concentrate	Exhausted Night sweats			Hot flush	Night sweats
Dragged myself to work Row at work	Mary mentions Dr Wang – he helped her	Very busy with the kids at home	Too tired to cook Jim angry	Visit Chinese doctor	Decided to take up yoga	Ann phones – has boyfriend happy now	Treatment seems to have helped bleeding already
All night	Poor	Better	Disturbed	Better	Good	Better	All night
	Dream of dragons				Meeting the Snake Woman in a cave		
Cheese sandwich and donut Cola drink	No lunch Chinese takeaway	Big lunch + pre-drinks + wine	Fish & chips			Salad lunch	Pasta Tried porridge for breakfast
sleeping pill	Tried camomile tea – yuck	More camomile tea		Camomile tea Acupuncture	Yunnan Baiyao Guipiwan shi Chuan Da Bu Wan	Y.B. G. SCDBW	Y.B. G. SCDBW

Food

The food you eat has a great deal to do with your sense of well-being and the moods and symptoms you experience at the time of menopause. Food allergy can be a trigger for hot flushes, depression, skin itching, aches and pains and many other conditions. Without keeping a record, few of us know just how many drinks we consume in a day (especially with sugar and caffeine which is found in tea, coffee, chocolate and many soft drinks). Caffeine is a trigger not only for hot flushes but also for mastitis (breast inflammation) and in addition it has an insidious effect on calcium absorption (important in the prevention of osteoporosis). The hidden sugar and salt content of foods can create symptoms which mimic those of menopause. Many herb teas have a medicinal effect and should also be monitored. If they are being taken specifically for this effect, then they should be entered under treatments.

Treatments

Unless a record is kept, it is impossible to see whether treatment for the physical or psychological symptoms of menopause is working, or indeed whether it is creating further problems with side-effects. Many people find, for instance, that HRT has the side-effect of inducing nausea, and natural progesterone may cause spotting when it is first used. All 'treatments' should be included, especially those such as acupuncture, massage and exercise. It is important to remember that natural treatments may take longer to 'work' and the effects may only become apparent over weeks or months.

Working with the diary information

Once you have kept a record over a month or two, patterns should begin to appear and the triggers become obvious. Using a coloured felt-tip pen to underline important items can help to bring the picture to life. If connections between the different boxes occur once or even twice, it may be coincidence. But if they appear regularly they will be significant. You will identify areas of your life that need revision and it may be necessary to reframe some underlying beliefs. You may find it helpful to avoid particular foods or activities in the week leading up to a period, or to take herbal medicines to deal with problems like insomnia at this time. You can learn to attune to the rhythm of your own sexuality, entering a more fulfilling sexual phase.

In the sample page (which is a 'worst case' scenario), you can see that there is evidence of prolonged and heavy bleeding which is linked to extreme tiredness and irritability. (A serious medical condition has already been ruled out.) This leads to additional stress at work and difficult family relationships. Her diet is not good and there is a possibility that both alcohol and coffee may be linked to hot flushes and night sweats. Chocolate binges affect her blood sugar levels. As sleeping pills leave her tired all day, she tries *camomile* tea which helps her sleep. On day seven of her cycle she visits a Chinese doctor. He diagnoses an energy imbalance involving the spleen. He prescribes one phial of *Yunnan Baiyao* taken over three days to stop the bleeding and two Chinese formulas to strengthen the spleen and stop bleeding and to nourish energy and blood. These will be taken daily for a month and will also help the depression. He gives her acupuncture to balance her energies, calm stress and help her sleep. In the weeks to come, the outcome of treatment will be a return to normal bleeding and far less tiredness and depression, which will in turn lead to a better quality of life.

If you are keeping an expanded journal, then the therapeutic effects will quickly become apparent and you may wish to continue it even after menopause. Such a journal is helpful if you are having any form of counselling or if you belong to a menopause self-help group, as it provides a starting point for sharing your experience. However, you can keep this journal as private as you wish, using it to record your own personal transition through this major life change.

III: Body

*Change is water flowing under bridges
a leaf carried by the flood to fortune or to oblivion*

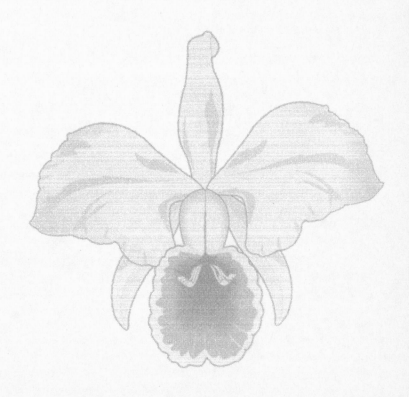

Hormone Replacement Therapy (HRT)

As orthodox medicine has come to believe that menopause is a hormonal deficiency — that is, a disease — rather than a naturally occurring process, doctors supplement hormone levels by the artificial replacement of the 'missing' hormones. These hormones may be 'natural' or synthetic. Initially oestrogen alone was prescribed, until an increased incidence of cancer was noted. Oestrogen was then prescribed in conjunction with progestogen to overcome this problem. Some doctors now believe that oestrogen dominance is the cause of menopausal symptoms and certain post-menopausal conditions, and that supplementation with natural progesterone may be required. There is evidence to suggest that an increased incidence of cancer may accompany prolonged use of HRT.[1] A recent study showed that an extra two women in a thousand, rising to six women in a thousand after ten years, would develop breast cancer when on HRT. You may live an average of $3^1/_2$ years longer on HRT.[2] There is also evidence to suggest you are at twice the normal risk of a blood clot (thrombosis) in the first year of HRT treatment.[3] Recommendations for length of use vary from two years to 'life'.

There are medical conditions which make HRT unsafe in the opinion of many doctors, although other doctors believe that even in these cases the benefit of HRT outweighs the high risk factor. Breast cancer and uterine cancer are generally regarded as absolute contraindications and many authorities recommend avoiding HRT if breast cancer runs in the family or if you have a personal history of heart attacks, strokes or pulmonary embolism (blood clots in the lungs). HRT can seriously exaggerate endometriosis (an abnormal but benign proliferation of the lining of the womb into sites where it does not normally occur) as bleeding can occur at non-uterine sites even after hysterectomy. HRT may make fibroids bigger. Left to themselves, fibroids naturally shrink after menopause and endometriosis no longer causes bleeding and other problems but this is not the case if HRT is given. HRT should not be taken within one year of an acute attack of hepatitis, or at all if suffering from hepatitis C. High blood pressure, smoking and obesity should all be reduced before starting HRT. It is admitted by the manufacturers of HRT that oestrogen may exacerbate otosclerosis (a type of middle ear deafness), multiple sclerosis, systemic lupus erythematosus, porphyria, melanoma, asthma, migraine, diabetes and epilepsy.

▶ *Fact File*

HRT is used both as preventive medicine and to alleviate the symptoms of menopause such as hot flushes and dry vagina.

▶ *Four main types of HRT:*

Tablets: Usually supplied in four-week packs consisting of oestrogen, taken once a day for 25 days, supplemented by progestogen on days 16 to 25. Days 26-30/31, no tablets taken. Hormones are absorbed via the digestive tract.

Patches: Used like band-aids on the lower abdomen, changed every three or four days. Hormones are absorbed through the skin.

Implants: Placed under the skin under local anaesthetic and remain in place for six months.

Creams: Used for local applications to offset vaginal dryness or urinary tract inflammation.

Most types of HRT produce a monthly bleed.

Most effective for: hot flushes and night sweats, vaginal dryness, anxiety and insomnia, confusion and memory loss.

Claimed to prevent: osteoporosis and heart disease (but recent research suggests otherwise — see references).

Possible side-effects of HRT: withdrawal bleeding, irregular vaginal bleeding, nausea, vomiting, breast/ovarian/uterine cancers, gallstones, strokes, thrombosis, elevated blood pressure, abdominal cramps, bloating, jaundice, premenstrual-like syndrome, vaginal candidiasis, skin rashes, changes in cervical erosion/secretions, breast tenderness/enlargement/secretion, chloasma or melasma (abnormal pigmentation or rash on the face), loss of scalp hair, hirsutism, steepening of corneal curvature, intolerance to contact lenses, headaches, migraine, dizziness, mental depression, chorea (St Vitus Dance), changes in weight, oedema (water retention), changes in libido, leg cramps, glucose intolerance, hypercalcaemia (high blood calcium). Patches: blistering or redness of skin.

Increased risk of: breast cancer (2 women in 1000 rising to 6 women after 10 years), ovarian cancer (70% after ten years according to one study[2]) and uterine cancer (on oestrogen: 4.5 to 13.9 times more likely), gallstones (2.5 times higher), stroke, thrombosis (3.5 times more likely, rising to 7 times at 1.25 mg; greatest risk: short-term users[4]), elevated blood pressure.

Contraindications: breast or uterine cancer, previous heart attack or stroke, abnormal blood fats, thromboembolic disease such as deep vein thrombosis or pulmonary embolism, breast dysplasia, acute liver disease, hepatitis C infection, high blood pressure, heavy smoking, obesity, fibroids, endometriosis, vaginal bleeding of unknown cause (requires immediate investigation).

Safety: Current HRT research findings are contradictory to say the least but many raise serious questions as to safety. One study will 'prove' what another study 'disproves'. If in doubt, consult the latest literature (the journal *What Doctors Don't Tell You* and medical journals carry up-to-date scientific study results).

HRT is not a contraceptive. If you are still ovulating, then you need to take contraceptive measures. If normal periods have ceased, then contraception should be continued for at least six to twelve months to prevent pregnancy.

Many menopausal 'symptoms' return when HRT is discontinued as the body's natural processes of adapting to changing hormone levels cannot function whilst on HRT.

Taking HRT can increase the body's need for vitamin B_6 (found in wholemeal bread, whole grains, milk, yeast, egg yolk, rice and bran).

Researchers have found that a large proportion of women discontinue use within the first few months without informing their doctor, due to unacceptable side-effects.

Premarin™, a 'natural' HRT comes from pregnant mare's urine. Throughout pregnancy the mares are tied in stalls, unable to move. The foals are often killed at birth.

HRT should be stopped if the following conditions develop: Pregnancy, breast or uterine cancer, thrombophlebitis, thromboembolism, jaundice, migraine, visual disturbance, increased blood pressure.

Patients with the following conditions should be carefully monitored:

Cardiac or renal dysfunction, endometriosis, breast nodules, fibrocystic breast disease

HRT should be discontinued prior to surgery or prolonged immobilisation

Coming off HRT: wherever possible, cut down the dosage gradually to allow the body's natural hormone production to take over.

After menopause, left to itself, the body produces the sex hormone oestrone from adrenal gland secretions. HRT interferes with this natural process.

References

1   Study by Imperial Cancer Research Fund's Epidemiology Unit at Oxford, quoted in *The Lancet,* October 1997, and several other studies
2   Study by the New England Medical Centre and The Tufts University School of Medicine, Boston. Quoted in *Daily Mail,* 10 April 1997.
3   *BMJ,* March 1997
4   *The Lancet,* 1996, 348:97780 and 98183

See also:

WDDTY, Vol. 4 No. 9 p. 1 and Vol. 6 No. 4 p. 6 (*see Further Reading*)
Menopause Matters, Judy Hall & Robert Jacobs. Element Books, Shaftesbury, 1994
What Doctors Don't Tell You, Lynne McTaggart. Thorsons, London, 1996

Is HRT for me?

If you are physically healthy and are suffering from hot flushes, night sweats, dry vagina, insomnia and unexplained anxiety or depression, or have had your ovaries removed, then HRT could well help in the short term (but see contraindications). Most doctors will prescribe HRT on these grounds or as a preventive measure if osteoporosis or heart disease run in your family.

Many doctors now routinely prescribe HRT for their menopausal patients, regardless of lack of 'symptoms' or medical indications. It is considered to be a preventive medicine worth giving 'just in case' — although few doctors are aware of the contradictory results of research trials.

Many women find the side-effects of HRT, such as nausea and withdrawal bleeding, unacceptable. Most doctors insist that nausea and other digestive tract upsets will disappear given time, and many suggest doubling the dose if the HRT does not appear to be working immediately. There are new forms of HRT available which minimise bleeding (but see the list of side-effects in the FactFile). Nevertheless, there are recognised contraindications to HRT (reasons not to take it).

▶ *ToDo*

▶ ***Is it safe for me to take HRT?***

Tick the box if you have any of the following conditions:

Cancer of the breast ☐

Cancer of the uterus ☐

Other hormone-dependent cancers ☐

Vaginal bleeding of unknown cause ☐

Endometriosis ☐

Pregnancy ☐

Liver disease including hepatitis C ☐

Active thrombophlebitis (vein inflammation) ☐

Thromboembolic disorder (blood clots) ☐

Rotor or Dubin-Johnson syndrome (congenital liver disorder) ☐

Severe cardiac or renal disease ☐

Previous heart attack ☐

Previous stroke ☐

Allergy to HRT constituents ☐

Obesity ☐

Fibroids ☐

Strong family history of breast cancer ☐

Abnormal blood fats ☐

Do you smoke heavily? ☐

Otosclerosis (a form of middle-ear deafness) ☐

Multiple sclerosis ☐

Systemic lupus erythematosus (SLE) ☐

Porphyria (congenital metabolic illness) ☐

Melanoma (skin cancer) ☐

Asthma ☐

Migraine ☐

Diabetes ☐

Epilepsy ☐

If you tick one or more of the boxes you should seriously question, and discuss with your doctor, the advisability of taking HRT and explore the possibility of alternative treatments with suitably qualified practitioners.

If you have any of the contraindications to HRT, then homoeopathy or flower essences are the safest alternative for you.

▶ ### Am I suffering from HRT side-effects?

Tick the box if you suffer from:

Nausea ☐

Indigestion ☐

Withdrawal bleeding ☐

PMS ☐

Headaches ☐

Candida ☐

Cramps ☐

Depression ☐

Disturbed sleep ☐

'Not feeling right' ☐

All of the above can be side-effects of HRT.

▶ ### Do I actually need HRT?

The only way to ascertain whether or not you need HRT, or natural hormones, is to have the appropriate medical tests to establish your hormonal status. Even then, you need to bear in mind that what the medical profession now considers to be a deficiency may actually be a natural, perfectly balanced state for this stage of your life. If a medical consultant tells you that you are 'hormone deficient', it is worth getting a further opinion from someone qualified in the complementary field who may well interpret the test results differently.

Unfortunately, because HRT has been hailed in the press over the last few years as 'the panacea for all ills', 'the pill for eternal youth', 'the only way to prevent osteoporosis and dowager's hump', 'a preventive medicine for heart disease and stroke', and other such extravagant claims (for which there is less and less supporting evidence), a generation of women have simply gone along with their doctor's recommendations and taken HRT regardless of whether they really needed it or not. Some women definitely feel better on HRT, others do not. But they are afraid to come off HRT because of the dire consequences that might follow, or so they are told. Other women have been told that they need HRT 'for life'. If you are one of these women, you may need to ask yourself some questions.

▶ *ToDo*

Tick the boxes that apply to you:	*Yes*	*No*
Do I actually have a hormone imbalance?	☐	☐
Do I feel good on HRT?	☐	☐
Did I have any symptoms?	☐	☐
Do I have any symptoms now?	☐	☐
Was there a medical reason such as hysterectomy?	☐	☐
Am I afraid of looking older?	☐	☐
Have I considered the evidence carefully?	☐	☐
Is there a safer alternative I could use?	☐	☐
Do I actually want to remain suspended in menopause or do I want to move on?	☐	☐

If you feel good, if your body is not rejecting the treatment, then the HRT may well be beneficial to you in the short term. However, if you feel unwell or 'not right' but persevere because you feel you ought to or because you found hot flushes or other symptoms unbearable, then it would be sensible to look at alternative options. It would also be useful to look at questions such as 'Are you afraid of getting old?'

Have you been scared by propaganda about osteoporosis and other relevant matters? If you are afraid of getting old, then the Mood and Mind sections of this book will help you. If you are concerned about osteoporosis, then it would be as well to investigate current nutritional thinking before you make your decision — see the section on osteoporosis. If you feel you need help in moving through menopause, then the natural remedies and mind/feelings-orientated approach outlined in this book can help you.

If you have had a surgically induced menopause following removal of the ovaries, then you are more likely to need and benefit from hormone replacement than someone who has not.

Natural Remedies

Natural alternatives to HRT

There are many natural alternatives to HRT, few of which have any side-effects or contraindications. *You are strongly advised to consult an appropriately qualified practitioner before embarking on a course of natural hormone replacement therapy or menopausal treatment* — and to check out exactly how 'natural' commercially produced plant hormones are.

Homoeopathy, acupuncture, acupressure, herbs and flower essences all act on menopausal symptoms with a gentle touch.

Flower essences are made by steeping flowers in spring water and then preserving the infused water in brandy. Their use in medicine dates back to ancient Egypt and beyond. As in homoeopathy, the energetic and vibrational signature of the flower is transferred to the essence. This is the highest and most refined expression of the healing properties of plants. Flower essences work on all levels. They can treat emotional and mental dis-ease but also work on the physical level and bodily function. They rarely have side-effects.

Acupuncture and acupressure work by balancing the energies along meridians in the body. Appropriate points are stimulated either with a needle or by finger pressure.

Homoeopathy is an energy-based system of medicine that is founded on the principle of 'like cures like'. A minute amount of a substance which would, in large quantities, produce the same symptoms as the disease being treated is prepared in such a way that the energy imprint only is administered (known as a potency). The remedies are diluted to such an extent that no molecules of the actual substance are present. Samuel Hahnemann, the founder of modern homoeopathy, based his treatment on the ideas of Paracelsus, a renowned Renaissance physician and alchemist. He believed that as the material substance was diluted out of the remedy, so a spiritual force entered into it. (This is a useful analogy for menopause. As a woman moves beyond the physical activities of child-rearing that tie her to the material world, so a space is created for a move towards the spirit.) There is evidence to support the theory that, at an electromagnetic level, homoeopathic remedies differ from one another even whilst they are identical on ordinary chemical analysis.

There are two types of homoeopathy, classical and complex. Classical homoeopathy uses single remedies, especially the 'constitutional remedy'. The constitutional remedy is based on Hahnemann's observation that some people behave as though they are chronically poisoned by a particular substance, showing symptoms that fit a specific remedy. A constitutional remedy is deep-acting, working on the mental as well as the physical level. It needs to be prescribed by a homoeopathic practitioner, as do other remedies, since the remedy is matched to the whole person, not to a 'disease'.

Complex homoeopathy uses remedies in combination to detoxify and cleanse the system as well as to treat disorders. Remedies act on particular organs and conditions, so this system is less holistic than classical homoeopathy. However, the complex homoeopaths point out that we are under an increasing toxic load from pesticides, pollution, cigarettes and drugs (including medically prescribed substances), which interfere with the working of the classical remedies, and so they add herbs to the mix to overcome this.

In homoeopathy, a 'healing crisis' may be instigated where symptoms worsen rapidly. This is a very good sign that the remedy is the correct one and will work. Stopping the remedy for a few days and then starting again will alleviate the symptoms (probably for good).

Apart from a few useful 'first aid remedies', homoeopathic remedies need to be prescribed by a practitioner. Flower essences can, however, be used as appropriate without the need to consult anyone.

Herbs and homoeopathy have a long history of use as menopausal medicine. The effects are rarely scientifically studied and documented because the people doing research in this field are usually the drug companies who are looking for a chemical constituent that they can patent and make money from. However, herbs work through the interaction of all the parts of the plant, not just an isolated ingredient, which makes them safer than patented chemicals. As we have seen, homoeopathy works on a 'like treats like' basis in which such minute dilutions of substances are used that only an energy trace remains, so there is nothing to patent. Many plants contain oestrogen-like substances or oestrogen precursors, which means they function like an organic HRT.

Natural hormones are derived from plants. They have a similar action to that of the hormones found in the body. (They should not be confused with synthetic hormones which may be made from the same source but have their molecular structure altered.) They combine with the same receptors as the body's own hormones, but may not activate them in the same way. Thus the plant-derived hormones may not have the same risks attached to them as synthetic 'human' hormones such as oestrogen and progestogen.

Herbs may be obtained in pill form but many are taken as infusions, tinctures or decoctions. An infusion is made by pouring boiling water on the dried or fresh herb, a tincture is prepared by soaking the herb in alcohol, and a decoction by boiling the herb in water.

If you have a medical condition that precludes the use of HRT, then homoeopathy, Chinese medicine or flower essences are the most appropriate treatment for you.

Healing challenge

Natural remedies may precipitate a healing challenge — a period when you feel much worse. It is a good sign! Simply stop taking the remedy for a few days and then restart. Your symptoms should then clear. If they do not, consult your practitioner. You may also find it helpful to work through the sections on Mood and Mind. Healing challenges usually occur when toxins present in the body start to be flushed out.

▶ *Fact File*

▶ *Flower essences*

The following flower essences appear to have a similar effect to progesterone and hence would be useful in cases of oestrogen dominance. They can be taken singly or in combination:

Correa (LE)

Golden Waitsia (LE)

Pale Sundew (LE)

Purple Eremophilia (LE)

Wallflower Donkey Orchid (LE)

Yellow Leschenaultia (LE)

Hounds Tongue (Californian)

Old Man Banksia (Bush)

Femin Essence (Bush) harmonises any imbalances during menopause. It allows a woman to discover and feel good about her own body and beauty.

DTR 53 Menopause Flower & Gems Remedy (Him)

Menopause Aid Formula 22 (Him)

Women's Hormonal Harmoniser (Shell) rebalances hormones and aids against feeling misunderstood and out of sorts. Take for 6 days only (6 drops under tongue twice a day). Then wait 3 months before repeating for another 6 days if necessary.

▶ *Phytoestrol* (plant hormones)

Rhubarb and hops contain an oestrogen-like hormone known as phytoestrol. Other sources of phytoestrol are anise, celery, fennel, ginseng, alfalfa, red clover and liquorice. Soya beans and soya products, such as miso and tofu, are also a good source of oestrogen. Including these foods in your diet can help counteract oestrogen deficiency.

Plant hormones are available as tablets containing 4 mg of rhubarb root and 90 mg of hops under the name of Phytoestrol. Naturopath Harald Gaier says that Phytoestrol both treats menopausal symptoms and alleviates withdrawal symptoms for women coming off HRT. So far, no side-effects are known. For mild menopausal symptoms, dosage is one tablet after breakfast and one after supper. For more severe symptoms, the dose is doubled. Treatment should continue for several months under the supervision of a qualified herbalist.[1]

According to Dr David Smallbone of Higher Nature it is believed that extract of Mexican yam, as a tablet, capsule or cream, may act as a phytoestrogen providing a weak dose of oestrogen. This may be useful to supplement the natural progesterone manufactured from wild yam and available as a cream (see below).

▶ *Natural progesterone cream*

Natural progesterone, produced as a cream, is synthesised from a plant source sometimes called *wild yam*. The hormone is claimed to be identical to that produced by the ovaries and is known as natural progesterone to differentiate it from synthetic progestogen or progestin, which may have serious side-effects (see below). The position with regard to natural progesterone is far from clear. Many preparations such as tablets, capsules and creams made from wild yam (*Dioscorea Villosa* or *Mexicana*) are available which purport to contain progesterone. However, there is no evidence to show that wild yam can be converted by the body into progesterone (although it can act as a weak phytoestrogen — see above). The conversion has to be done by synthesis in a laboratory. To ensure that what you are using actually is natural progesterone, it is essential to purchase the cream from a reputable source and to use it under the guidance of an experienced practitioner.

Although many users highly recommend natural progesterone cream, the medical profession has been slow to endorse the product. In America and Europe it is available over the counter. In the UK it can be purchased as a 'cosmetic cream' or is available on prescription.

Natural progesterone is appropriate when your body is still producing a high level of oestrogen but is not producing sufficient progesterone. It counteracts oestrogen dominance. It would be sensible to have a hormone test to establish whether you are indeed deficient in progesterone before using natural progesterone.

Dr John Lee and several other researchers[2] who have been working with natural progesterone for at least 15 years have found no side-effects except perhaps for some spotting in the first month or two. In an article on natural progesterone *What Doctors Don't Tell You*[3] reported side-effects. However, it was later admitted that these were the side-effects of Gestone, an injectable progestogen synthetically produced from sisal fibre[4], not Mexican yam. They did not specifically relate to natural progesterone cream. Some authorities believe that artificially high levels of progestogen may lead to an increased risk of breast cancer but Dr Lee contends that natural progesterone actually helps to prevent cancer and reports considerable improvement in fibrocystic breast disease. In a retrospective study over thirty years, researchers at Johns Hopkins University found that women who were progesterone-deficient had a 5.4 times higher incidence of breast cancer and a 10 times higher incidence of death from cancers of all kinds.[5] Unlike HRT, natural progesterone does not exacerbate fibroids. Dr Lee found that these shrank significantly.

There are currently two studies being run at Chelsea & Westminster Hospital, London, on the effects of using progesterone-containing creams in menopause, and further trials are planned, so information on this subject will continue to grow.

Before you use natural progesterone cream, a simple test administered by a doctor at the appropriate stage of your menstrual cycle can check whether you are lacking progesterone. It is also possible to check the body's progesterone level by a saliva test.[6]

Dosage: the manufacturers of natural progesterone cream should supply guidance on usage which must be followed. It is taken as part of a cyclic process — normally for 21 days from the first day of your period (or the first day of the month if you are no longer menstruating), followed by a seven-day interval. It is rubbed, on a rotating basis, into areas of thin skin, such as the inner elbow, the wrists, backs of the knees etc. It should always be used under the supervision of a qualified practitioner. Check content carefully, as this will affect the dosage.

> Natural hormones need to be taken cyclically. Follow your practitioner's guidance.

▶ Wild yam extract

Various wild yam creams, capsules and tablets are available (see Resources). They do not necessarily contain natural progesterone and may act as a weak phytoestrogen. *Endau*, a wild yam extract containing natural progesterone and a DHEA analogue, is said to combine the benefits of progesterone and DHEA without side-effects. Endau can be applied topically during a hot flush.

▶ **DHEA** *(Dehydroepiandosterone)*

Extravagant claims are made for DHEA which it is suggested may be a 'Fountain of Youth', one of the greatest discoveries of the twentieth century and a cure-all for many diseases.[7] It is claimed that the only side-effects are beneficial ones, although mild abnormalities in blood sugar metabolism can occur when high doses are given, and acne or a slight increase in hair growth on arms and legs have been reported. There may also be initial breakthrough bleeding until oestrogen levels stabilise.

DHEA, a steroid hormone, occurs naturally in the body. It is produced mainly in the adrenal glands and is utilised in the manufacture of sex hormones. The amount of DHEA in the body dramatically declines with age. Typically, in women aged fifty, the blood level of DHEA is down 50%, and by seventy it has dropped to 31%. Low levels have been linked to cancer, osteoporosis, ageing, heart disease, immuno-deficiency, obesity, Alzheimers and rheumatoid arthritis.

DHEA is available as Youthinol, extracted from Mexican wild yam and further processed in the laboratory. The manufacturers claim that it is an analogue — a biologically usable compound — rather than the precursor found in rival products.

Dosage: One or more tablets twice daily as instructed. A low maintenance dose may be required after initial treatment.

▶ **Folliculinum** *(homoeopathically diluted and energised)*

A potentised form of synthetic oestrogen, Folliculinum, can be regarded as homoeopathic HRT. It suits women who feel drained and who have an irregular cycle with flooding. The typical picture is a hypersensitive woman who has lost her sense of herself and who feels dominated by another (often the husband). It is helpful in panic attacks and anxiety and also for hot flushes accompanied by night sweats with restlessness.

Folliculinum can also be used for treating adverse reactions to HRT and associated effects.

▶ *Sepia*

Another homoeopathic remedy, Sepia is a hormonal treatment *par excellence*. It is also helpful in depression. Sepia is made from the ink of cuttlefish, and Sepia patients often look as though they are under a black cloud. They wish to escape from the burden of family commitments. Prone to perspire easily, Sepia patients are helped by exercise and may be fond of dancing. Sepia should be given under the direction of a homoeopath as it may be needed in high potency.

▶ *She Oak*

An Australian Bush Flower essence, She Oak comes from the Aboriginal healing tradition. It is made from one of the first trees ever to evolve on Earth. Its globular female flower heads resemble the fallopian tubes waiting to catch eggs from the ovaries and one of its primary uses is in female infertility. It regulates and rebalances the production of reproductive hormones, especially where there is an irregular menstrual cycle. She Oak also helps to regulate water within the body and so may be useful in cases of water retention or overly dry conditions.

▶ *Agnus Castus*

Agnus Castus has a long history of use as a medicine. In classical times it was strewn by Athenian matrons in their beds. It was also used in the rites of Demeter, the Eleusinian mysteries. In medieval times, monks would use the ground-up seeds as a type of pepper because it helped them to be celibate — hence its name Monks Pepper or Chaste Tree. Fortunately it has a different effect on women.

Agnus Castus has a normalising effect on hormone production, especially that of progesterone. It contains oestrogen-like substances and so acts as an organic hormone replacement therapy.

Its action is twofold and opposite (amphoteric). In men, it is anaphrodisiac, in women aphrodisiac. These effects are related to its oestrogenic properties.

It is excellent for hot flushes, a dry vagina, breast tenderness or mastitis, PMS, digestive problems and depression, and may strengthen bones.

The berries are the active part of the plant and are used as a tincture (1-2 ml) or dried and ground (3-6 gm) three times a day (capsules are available). It is sold as Agnacast in most health food shops and is ideal for women who cannot tolerate medically prescribed HRT. Agnus Castus is also available in homoeopathic potency which is useful for women who have contraindications to HRT.

The effect of Agnus Castus may take up to three months to establish itself, so it is appropriate to take it for a period of up to six months. If symptoms recur, then the herb can be used again after a short break.

Caution: Side-effects have been reported following the use of Agnus Castus by well women.[8] These are rare but it may be preferable to take Agnus Castus as a homoeopathic preparation under the direction of a qualified practitioner.

▶ ***Red Sage*** *Salvia officinalis*

This herb has long been associated with women. Medieval astrologers assigned rulership of it to Venus, the planet of love, and it is known to have been used in ancient times.

Pharmacologically, Salvia has a number of active ingredients, amongst them minerals, vitamins and oestrogen-like substances. It regulates hormone imbalance and is drying and antiseptic in nature.

Salvia is excellent for hot flushes with profuse sweating, and also night sweats, as its drying action reduces perspiration considerably. It is also helpful in cases of excessive or prolonged bleeding. It should not be used, however, if the vagina is dry as it will exacerbate this condition. Salvia is also a natural tranquilliser and will ease anxiety and depression, and aid restful sleep. Its anti-inflammatory properties relieve aches and pains in the joints. Sage tea can eliminate nausea and flatulence.

As the herb can be grown on a window sill, it is a useful self-help remedy. Two or three leaves in hot water make an excellent calming tea. An infusion can be made from 5-10 gm of the leaves and taken twice daily or sipped during hot flushes or night sweats. Alternatively, 2-4 ml of the tincture can be taken three times a day.

Contraindication: Do not use if the vagina is dry.

▶ ### *False Unicorn Root (Helonias)* Chamaelirium luteum

False Unicorn Root is from the healing tradition of the North American Indians who use it as a female reproductive tonic. As it contains oestrogen precursors, the body converts it into oestrogen. It regularises and balances hormone function.

It is excellent for menstrual irregularities and urogenital problems, especially where the presenting symptom is a dragging ache in the lower abdomen. It also kills worms or parasites. Dosage: 3-9 gm of the root prepared as an infusion or tea, or 2 ml of the tincture, taken three times a day.

Warning: Emetic if used in large quantities.

▶ ### *Black Cohosh* Cimicifuga racemosa

Black Cohosh is also from the North American Indian tradition. Containing oestrogens, it normalises the female reproductive system, and is a powerful relaxant.

It is particularly useful where the menopause is accompanied by arthritis, muscular pain, anxiety or mental tension. It also reduces hot flushes and eases stress. It was traditionally used to prevent prolapse of the uterus.

One teaspoonful of the dried root is boiled with one cup of water for 10-15 minutes. This is then drunk three times a day. Alternatively, 2-4 ml of tincture may be taken three times a day.

Contraindication: Do not use in cases of heavy bleeding or flooding.

▶ **Camomile** *Matricaria chamomilla*

According to the Anglo-Saxons, Camomile was one of nine sacred herbs presented to humanity by the god Woden. It has long been used as a gynaecological herb, being well known to the Romans. Camomile contains glycosides, which have a sedative action, and components with a hormonal action. It is also a source of readily absorbable calcium.

It is an excellent sedative and relaxant and is frequently used for menopause accompanied by anxiety, stress and insomnia. It is also useful for painful periods and mastitis, and is a uterine tonic.

Camomile tea is readily available in supermarkets and health food stores. Taken at night, it will prevent sleeplessness. Therapeutically, 6-12 gm is taken as an infusion.

▶ **Motherwort** *Leonurus cardiaca*

The ancient Greeks used Motherwort to treat anxiety in pregnant women, hence its name. The medieval herbalist Culpeper wrote: "There is no better herb to drive melancholy vapours from the heart, to strengthen it and make the mind cheerful, blithe and merry."

It has a regulatory action on the muscles of the uterus and vagina, and is often used for painful periods. It also has appreciable sedative and relaxing effects.

Motherwort is appropriate when menopause is accompanied by palpitations, nervousness, tension and night sweats. It can also help depression and insomnia. It will tone the uterus, bladder and vagina and is helpful in menstrual cramps.

Contraindication: Motherwort should not be used when there is menstrual flooding.

▶ **Beth Root** *Trillium erectum*

Prized by the North American Indians for its aphrodisiac effect, Beth Root contains a natural precursor of the female sex hormones. It has a tonic effect on the uterus and drying qualities which make it useful for arresting excessive uterine bleeding (for which a gynaecological opinion should always be sought). It is usually given in combination with **Golden Seal** (*Hydrastis canadensis*), an endocrine gland tonic with a powerful antibiotic effect. Beth Root should always be used under the direction of a qualified herbalist.

▶ **Dong Quai** *Angelica sinensis*

A fast-acting Chinese herb, Dong Quai is a hormone regulator and helps relieve many menopausal conditions including hot flushes, water retention, anxiety and depression. It is usually prescribed in combination with other herbs and should be taken under the direction of a Chinese practitioner or herbalist.

Other Natural Remedies for Menopausal Symptoms

▶ **Vitamin E**

Vitamin E helps to relieve hot flushes by stabilising oestrogen levels. It is best taken with **vitamin C** and **selenium** to aid absorption. Dose: 30-100 mg.

Contraindication: High blood pressure, diabetes, heart problems, cancer.

▶ **GLA** *(Gammalinoleic Acid)*

Starflower, Borage and **Evening Primrose Oils**

GLA can reduce menopausal symptoms, improve mood and energy, and keep the skin healthy. (There is three times the amount of GLA in Starflower Oil than in Evening Primrose.)

▶ **Dr Jacobs' Flower Essence Mixture**

Beemdkroon [otherwise known as **Field Scabious**] (Bloesem), **Willow** (Alaskan), **Jacob's Ladder** (Alaskan) and **Sunflower** (Alaskan). Taken together, these essences relieve hot flushes and general menopausal symptoms.

Remedies for hot flushes

▶ **Mulla Mulla** *(Bush)*

Mulla Mulla grows in the hottest part of the Australian desert and is superb for 'hot' conditions such as sunburn, hot flushes and raised temperature. A few drops taken every few minutes will quickly ease a hot flush.

▶ **Belladonna**

Belladonna is an excellent 'first aid remedy' for flushing or raised temperature. Homoeopathic Belladonna is particularly useful where hot flushes are accompanied by sweating, congestion and redness of the face. (Take in 6x or 30x potency. Higher potencies should be prescribed by a homoeopath).

▶ **Sage** *(Salvia)*

Salvia tincture is used in homoeopathy for hot flushes which move from the chest upwards. Dose: 7-10 drops in water at night, increasing to 20 drops if necessary.

▶ **Lachesis**

The venom of the most poisonous snake on earth, the bushmaster, Lachesis is used in non-toxic homoeopathic dilution. It is an appropriate remedy for hot flushes accompanied by palpitations and headache, with a feeling of constriction around the throat, or choking fits, and sudden rushes of blood to the head. Specific indication for Lachesis: inability to tolerate anything tight around the neck. Helpful for heavy periods. Dosage: Under the direction of a homoeopath.

▶ **Glonoine** *(Glyceryl trinitrate)*

Glonoine is an allopathic drug which can also be given in homoeopathic dilution (thereby avoiding side-effects) where a throbbing headache accompanies the hot flush. Use under the direction of a homoeopath.

▶ **Amyl nitrite**

Another allopathic drug available in homoeopathic form, Amyl Nitrite aids hot flushes which come on suddenly, accompanied by headache, anxiety and palpitations. Use under the direction of a homoeopath.

▶ **Sulphur**

Sulphur is one of the 'constitutional remedies' of homoeopathy and needs to be tailored to the patient. A Sulphur patient is typically untidy, introspective and fond of sweet and fatty food.

▶ **Kali Carb** *(potassium carbonate)*

Another constitutional remedy, Kali Carb helps when hot flushes are accompanied by backache and weakness in the back and legs. Good for the ubiquitous menopausal symptoms of word loss, mistakes in speech, or sudden dyslexia when writing.

▶ **Calc Carb**

A further constitutional remedy, Calc Carb is a watery remedy and is helpful where flushes are accompanied by profuse perspiration. Clears water retention causing excess weight. A typical Calc Carb patient is pale and flabby, and feels the cold easily.

▶ ### *Aurum Metallicum*

This homoeopathic remedy aids hot flushes accompanied by depression and thoughts of suicide. At a potency of 30c, it can be a *'first aid essence'*.

▶ ### *Remedies for excessive bleeding*

Homoeopathic: *Sepia, Pulsatilla, Phosphorus*

Chinese: *Yunnan Bai Yao*

▶ ### *Remedies for insomnia*

Valerian (tincture or tablets)

Wild Lettuce

Camomile tea

Flower essences: mix: *Boronia, Crowea* and *Black-Eyed Susan* (Bush)

▶ ### *Remedy for lump in the throat*

Ignatia 6c

References

See *Menopause Matters,* Judy Hall & Robert Jacobs. Element Books, Shaftesbury, 1994

1   *WDDTY* Vol. 4 No. 9 p. 2 (*see Further Reading*)

2   *Passage to Power,* Leslie Kenton. Thorsons, 1996
     Natural Progesterone: A Nutrition Factsheet The Nutrition Line
     Natural Progesterone, J R Lee. BLL Publishing, California, 1993

3   *WDDTY* Vol. 6 No. 8 p. 853; *WDDTY* Vol. 6 No. 11 p. 8-9

4   Study quoted in *Some Basic Information About Progesterone*

5   Bio/Tech News: *The Hormone of Life. Natural Progesterone: a nutritional factsheet,* The Nutrition
     Line. Positive Health. April/May 1996
     Australian Bush Flower Essences Ian White. Findhorn Press, 1993

6   *Proof* Vol.1 (*see Further Reading*)

7   Personal correspondence to author referring to unspecified homoeopathic source

Self-Help: Acupressure

Acupressure, or shiatsu (the Japanese form), is available from qualified practitioners. However, it is also a useful self-help method of dealing with menopause. Acupressure involves stimulating an acupuncture point by massaging in a circular fashion with the finger or thumb (you can usually tell if you are on the right point because it hurts!). It is a useful first aid measure for hot flushes, headaches, insomnia and other conditions.

▶ *Daily regime*

Massage the points illustrated in the following diagrams at least once a day on both sides of the body to regulate hormone levels, boost energy, lessen hot flushes and calm the mind as required:

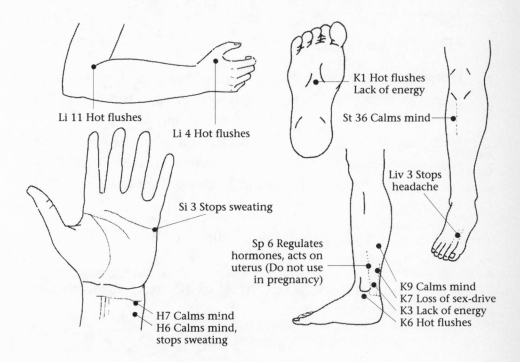

Fig 3: Daily regime

How Do I Decide Which is the Right Alternative Treatment for Me?

With so many alternatives available, it can sometimes be a daunting task to find exactly the right treatment. It is so often a matter of 'gut instinct' — the one that feels right (this is much easier when your intuition is working well and some of the exercises later in the book will help here). If you feel particularly drawn towards a therapy, try it out.

▶ *ToDo*

Tick the appropriate boxes:

	mild	severe
Are your symptoms	☐	☐

	yes	no
Have you had them a long time?	☐	☐
Are you otherwise healthy?	☐	☐

If your symptoms are severe, if you have had them a long time or if your health is generally poor, then you should consult a qualified practitioner. If your symptoms are mild or just beginning, then a good general introduction to herbal therapy would be **Agnacast** or **Motherwort** tincture or tablets taken for a month or two, depending on your symptoms. Or try **Dr Jacobs' Flower Essence Mixture**. The difference may be startling.

	yes	no
Do you suffer from any contraindications to HRT? (see page 81)	☐	☐

If yes, consult an experienced Chinese medicine, homoeopathic or flower essence practitioner.

	yes	no
Do you appear to be oestrogen dominant? (see page 23)	☐	☐

If you appear to be oestrogen dominant, then natural progesterone (wild yam) may help.

	yes	no
Is cost an important factor?	☐	☐

Flower essences are definitely the cheapest option. Some of the most useful for menopause are mentioned in this book. They cost only a few pounds each, last a long time and do not need a practitioner (although there are practitioners who can help). More and more books (see Further Reading) are available on the topic. The good ones are illustrated. A quick way to find a remedy is to look at the illustrations of flowers and see which one you are drawn to (you can mentally ask for guidance). Then look up the indications. At first sight, it may not always seem to have much relevance but it is always appropriate.

Homoeopathy is also one of the less costly options. Although you have to pay the practitioner's consultation fee, the remedies themselves are inexpensive.

Acupuncture treatments are not usually expensive. You do need them at reasonably frequent intervals, but acupuncture works quickly.

yes   no

Are you suffering from mental stress, pain, insomnia, ☐ ☐
lack of energy?

If yes, acupuncture or Chinese medicine are likely to be of help.

Can you bear needles? ☐ ☐

If no, choose acupressure or Chinese herbs rather than acupuncture.

Can you cope with strange and bitter tastes? ☐ ☐

If the answer to this one is no, herbs may not be for you, although they are increasingly available as pills, especially the tonic formulas.

A practitioner who is proficient in the use of the Vega Test Machine (see Resources, Noma) or a similar electro-diagnostic system would be able to test you for the most appropriate type of remedy, be this herbal, homoeopathic or even allopathic (HRT). A competent AK (Applied Kinesiology) practitioner could do the same.

Sexuality

Whilst there is absolutely no reason why sex should not continue to be enjoyed right through and after midlife change — and indeed may become much more pleasurable afterwards — loss of libido (lack of interest in sex) sometimes accompanies the menopause, as does dryness of the vagina. However, these two are not necessarily linked, nor are they specifically menopausal problems. Loss of libido almost always responds to a change of sexual partner and psychological factors may be involved (see Mind, page 193 onwards).

HRT is often prescribed for loss of libido, but not all cases respond to it, suggesting that oestrogen deficiency is not a primary cause of lack of interest in sex. Natural progesterone, on the other hand, has been found to aid the condition. A simple exercise performed twice a day can unlock your libido (see page 111). Australian Bush Flower Essences gently adjust any deep-seated feelings which may be inhibiting sexual drive and herbs can help maintain the correct hormonal balance. In Chinese medicine, loss of libido is seen as arising from an energetic imbalance within the body, an imbalance that can be corrected with acupuncture and herbs.

Dryness of the vagina may be caused by oestrogen deficiency but does not necessarily have to be treated with oestrogen, although oestrogen-containing creams are available if appropriate. Homoeopathic remedies, herbs and even using natural bio-yoghurt as a vaginal douche can help to overcome vaginal dryness and thinning (vaginitis). Over-the-counter creams are readily available from pharmacies: KY jelly has been used for years as a vaginal lubricant, while Replens is one of the newer ones. Nor is vaginal dryness an inevitable consequence of menopause.

▶ *FactFile*

Having an ongoing healthy sex life is the best prevention against sexual problems at menopause.

Menopausal women may need longer foreplay.

Loss of libido can be caused by medically prescribed drugs.

Androgens (male sex hormones such as testosterone) are sometimes implanted in women to overcome loss of libido. It can give rise to unwanted side-effects of masculinisation, increased growth of facial hair and permanent deepening of the voice.

▶ *Natural remedies for loss of libido*

Agnus Castus
Saffron (*Crocus sativus*) in small quantity added to food
Natural progesterone cream
Beth Root

Homoeopathy: *Sepia, Murex*
Chinese herbalism has many remedies but these need to be prescribed by a practitioner

▶ *Natural remedies to counteract dryness*

Bryonia (homoeopathic): take internally 6x twice daily
Motherwort (tincture): take internally 6-10 drops twice daily
Agnus Castus (tincture, tablets or homoeopathy): take internally
Calendula cream: apply to vagina internally
Aloe Vera: apply to vagina internally
Natural progesterone oil: apply externally

▶ *Australian Bush Flower remedies for vaginitis*

Dagger Hakea, Sturt Desert Rose, Billy Goat Plum

▶ *Remedy to counteract cystitis*

Cranberry juice

▶ *Remedy for vaginal discharge and non-specific cervical changes*

Pulsatilla 6x, twice daily

▶ ***Vaginal oestrogen cream*** *(Ortho-Dienestrol)*

Prescribed for a dry vagina. Oestrogen cream is absorbed by the walls of the vagina and carries the same risks as HRT, including endometrial cancer and possibly cervical, vaginal and liver cancers. Use of the treatment for over two years may cause a predisposition towards gallstones.

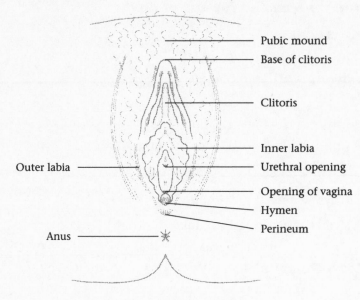

Pubic mound
Base of clitoris
Clitoris
Inner labia
Outer labia
Urethral opening
Opening of vagina
Hymen
Perineum
Anus

Fig 4: External female genitalia

Pleasuring yourself

Most girls are brought up with exhortations 'not to touch' (exactly what is rarely specified). Self-pleasuring — masturbation — is somehow seen as 'not nice', 'downright sinful' or 'dirty' (see Mind section). Teenagers often find out that masturbation is actually a pleasurable activity. Even so, many women continue to believe that it is not for them. However, masturbation has its benefits, especially in midlife. Quite apart from giving you pleasure, masturbation is a way of keeping your vagina healthy. If you do not have regular sexual stimulation, then it is more likely that you will suffer from dryness and thinning of the vaginal walls during or after menopause — conditions that make sex a painful experience. So using a vibrator or discovering the joys of masturbation can be therapeutic. It will keep the walls of the vagina lubricated and elastic.

If you have a partner, you can privately explore what pleasures you and share this knowledge later with your partner. Your sex life might improve quite dramatically (some men find the idea of women masturbating quite a turn-on; lesbian women tend to know all about masturbation already).

Be imaginative. Many women fantasise but often all the action takes place in the head. You can let your vagina join in the fun. Masturbation doesn't have to take place in bed. You may find that a warm bath is the ideal place for a bit of self-pampering with an aphrodisiac oil.

If you have never tried masturbation before, you may be surprised at how easy it is — and at the intense sensations you can experience this way. First of all, make sure you know where your clitoris is (not all women do — see the illustration). Then spend time exploring and experimenting. Use your fingers first. Do you like a light touch or a heavy one? Do you prefer to be inside or outside your vagina? Work around your clitoris. Try different positions for your hand and fingers: it is possible to stimulate several different parts of yourself at once. Use a vibrator if you wish. Remember to breathe — breath helps the sexual energy to circulate.

As you become more stimulated and move closer to orgasm, let your hand rest on your pubic mound. Your fingers then curl over your clitoris and into the vagina. With practice, you can involve your whole body in your orgasm. As the contractions of orgasm begin, have your finger at the base of the clitoris. Feel the energy move into the base of your spine. As orgasm continues, move your hand back slightly up the clitoris. At the same time, feel the energy moving up your spine. Continue to pull your hand back to the top of the clitoris. By then the energy will be pulsing right up your spine to the top of your head. Breathe out and let the energy flow right through your body to your fingers and toes. Multiple orgasm is easy this way — as each orgasm finishes, move your hand back to your starting point and, with a little gentle stimulation, you will be ready once again.

▶ *ToDo*

Do you actually know what your genital area looks like? If not, find a mirror and have a good look.

Tick the box if you are taking any of the following:

Tranquillisers ☐

Antidepressants ☐

Blood pressure tablets ☐

Beta-blockers ☐

Tablets for excessive bleeding ☐

All of the above can cause loss of libido

	yes	no
Can you reach orgasm?	☐	☐
With a partner?	☐	☐
Alone?	☐	☐
Have you tried it alone?	☐	☐
Do you feel you need more foreplay?	☐	☐
Do you always make love in the same position?	☐	☐
— in the same place?	☐	☐
Is there a new position you'd like to try?	☐	☐

If you cannot reach orgasm on your own, then you could be helped by appropriate counselling.

Boredom can be a major factor in loss of libido, as can lack of stimulation — emotional as well as physical.

Share with your partner exactly what turns you on and how you like to be stimulated. Experiment with new positions (try one that stimulates your clitoris or allows room for your partner's hands to do this). Insist on it.

Give your partner a massage — with no expectation as to sex.

Have a massage from your partner — with no expectation as to sex.

▶ *Awakening the libido*

Stand with your legs slightly apart and placed directly under your hips. Slowly move your hips in a wide circle going out to the right, to the front, out to the left, then to the back. Repeat ten times, then change direction. Do this night and morning for a least two weeks.

▶ *Toning exercise for the vagina and bladder*

This exercise strengthens the pelvic floor, preventing prolapse and incontinence as well as toning the vaginal muscles. With practice you will be able to contract different muscle groups at the front of the vagina and then around the anus. The best way to carry out this exercise at first is when you are on the loo so that you see the effect of contraction on the flow of urine. After that it can be done sitting, standing or lying down.

> Contract the muscles of the vagina and hold for a count of ten. Then relax. Repeat ten times. Practise several times a day.

> Once you have learnt how to do this exercise, it can be carried out at any time or in any place during the day.

Note: *as sexuality really cannot be separated from feelings and attitudes, see Mood and Mind chapters.*

Osteoporosis

Osteoporosis (thinning bones) can be a consequence of menopause but it does not have to be. It is not a menopausal disease. In some women it can occur before the menopause and some researchers believe that it has its roots in the mid-thirties. It is a 'silent disease' which only becomes apparent many years after its onset.

Osteoporosis occurs when, in normally mineralised bone, the overall volume of bone tissue per volume of bone is reduced. The bone is not deficient in calcium, but there is actually less bone present. That is, the bones become thin, honeycomb-like and prone to spontaneous fracture. This occurs when the natural process of bone breakdown and reabsorption takes place faster than new bone growth. Up to now osteoporosis could only be detected by an expensive bone-density scan, or was indicated by a history of spontaneous fractures. However, a new test being developed by University Diagnostics in Britain is under trial. It detects a bone degradation product in urine and will enable rapid and cheap recognition of the onset of osteoporosis. Another new test, the Achilles Plus, uses ultrasound to detect changes in the heelbone. As this is one of the first bones to lose density, early treatment will prevent further bone loss.

Osteoporosis is understood by most doctors to be a hormonal deficiency disease resulting from declining levels of oestrogen. It also occurs in progesterone-deficient women. Oestrogen slows down the breakdown and reabsorption of old bone. Progesterone stimulates the formation of new bone. At menopause, hormonal changes can affect the balance between the two processes and progesterone production in the body may cease, leaving oestrogen the dominant hormone. This means that bone breakdown will continue but bone replacement will not, resulting in the typically 'spongy', honeycombed bone of osteoporosis.

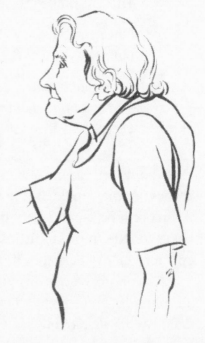

However, other subtle body processes also affect the utilisation of calcium and osteoporosis may be caused by a nutritional imbalance rather than a specifically hormonal one.[1] It has been shown that enzymes, lack of stomach acid, and vitamin and mineral deficiencies all play their part in osteoporosis. As diet, exercise, smoking and drinking, and cooking utensils can also play a part, osteoporosis should more correctly be called a lifestyle disease.

Fig 5: Typical osteoporosis posture

▶ *FactFile*

Not all post-menopausal women will suffer from osteoporosis. But this debilitating condition is increasing and one in three women now suffer from it.

Osteoporosis should be confirmed by the appropriate test before treatment to avoid unnecessary use of drugs.

More women die after a hip fracture than from cancer of the uterus, cervix and ovaries combined.

Osteoporosis can affect men as well as women.

Prolonged use of corticosteroids can cause osteoporosis.

▶ *Indications*

Reduced height ('shrinking')

'Dowager's hump'

Back and neck pain

Spontaneous fractures of wrist, hip and spine

Low bone density (Bone density is not apparent from external examination. It only shows on bone scans.)

▶ *Most effective preventive treatment*

Sufficient calcium intake and supporting minerals, especially in youth, to ensure peak bone density mass prior to menopause.

Good nutrition and a varied wholefood diet. (Restrict protein, salt, alcohol and caffeine intake.) Your total salt intake should not exceed 5g (1 teaspoonful) per day.

Sufficient, appropriate and regular exercise before, during and after menopause to maintain bone health. Whether or not you develop osteoporosis depends largely on the correct amount of exercise taken in youth.

The Chinese herb *He Shou Wu* is an excellent preventive and treatment.

Calcium is essential for maintaining bone mass. High intake of red meat, phosphorus (found in milk and cola drinks), and aluminium (contained in antacids, soya milk and some saucepans) can interfere with the absorption of calcium.

Vitamin D is essential for absorption of calcium. Fifteen minutes' daily exposure to sunshine enables the body to produce sufficient Vitamin D. A correct balance of magnesium, zinc, manganese, phosphorus and vitamins A and C is also essential for proper use of calcium, all of which should be found in a good, well varied wholefood diet. (If supplementation is indicated consult a nutritional practitioner.)

▶ *Calcium-rich foods*

Parmesan cheese	Sesame seeds	Tahini
Whole grains	Tuna	Sardines (with bones)
Salmon	Cheddar cheese	Carob powder
Spinach	Parsley	Broccoli
Tofu	Milk	Haricot & lima beans
Figs	Egg yolks	Blackstrap molasses
Yoghurt	Chick peas	Almonds
Cottage cheese	Rhubarb	Brazil nuts
Hazelnuts	Sea vegetables	Red kidney beans
Carbonated mineral water		

Calcium supplementation: The role of calcium supplementation in preventing osteoporosis is unclear. Different scientific studies have given conflicting results. Sufficient intake, combined with essential vitamins and minerals, through diet is recommended.

Researcher Dr John McLaren Howard[2] found that none of the women in his study had low calcium levels but they were deficient in the nutrients associated with bone development and in alkaline phosphatase, a bone enzyme. The lowest levels of alkaline phosphatase were found in women taking HRT for osteoporosis. Dr Guy Abraham[2] believes magnesium deficiency contributes to low alkaline phosphatase. Supplementing with magnesium showed an 11% increase in bone density over eight months.

▶ *Magnesium-rich foods*

Millet, Lima beans, brazil nuts, yoghurt, dark green vegetables

▶ *Exercise*

Regular isometric and weight-bearing exercise helps to prevent bone loss. Yoga, tai chi chuan, qigong, dancing, brisk walking, tennis, working with weights, cycling and carrying the shopping home instead of using the car are appropriate forms of exercise.

Excessive exercise and hard athletic or dance training can lead to osteoporosis.

Treatment

▶ *HRT*

Prevention of osteoporosis is the most cited reason for prescribing HRT. HRT is believed to prevent further bone loss. It does not rebuild new bone. Bone loss recommences and accelerates as soon as HRT is withdrawn. Authorities disagree as to the length of time HRT should be taken to prevent bone fractures in old age. Some recommend at least ten years and others believe that even this is not long enough.

▶ *Natural progesterone cream*

Natural progesterone cream is synthesised from Mexican Yam. The position on natural progesterone is far from clear. It is not yet licensed as a medicine but can be obtained on prescription. It is available for 'cosmetic purposes' without prescription. Some authorities recommend it highly; others are cautious, especially with regard to possible side-effects such as breast cancer — which advocates claim is prevented by natural progesterone.

Dr John Lee, who has been working with natural progesterone combined with nutrition and exercise since 1982, claims that not only does it halt bone loss but actually reverses it. He has seen a 10% increase in bone density within a year, followed by a 3-5% increase until bone density stabilised to that of a healthy 35-year-old.[4] None of the 67 women who participated in his three-year trial suffered from fractures due to osteoporosis during that period.

Natural progesterone cream is rubbed on large areas of thin skin such as the palms of the hands, wrists, neck and upper chest (rotation of sites is recommended) and is taken up by the fatty tissue before passing into the bloodstream. The manufacturer's instructions must be followed. Up to three months may elapse before effects are felt. Prolonged use is necessary to prevent osteoporosis.

Natural progesterone should be used under the guidance of a suitably qualified practitioner.

Wild or Mexican Yam extract is also available as oral preparations but there is no evidence to suggest that these have an effect on osteoporosis.

▶ **DHEA** *(Dehydroepiandosterone)*

This naturally occurring steroid hormone is produced in the body in the adrenal glands. It is one of the major hormonal building blocks. Studies have shown that women with the lowest levels of DHEA suffer the greatest bone-density loss and women with the highest levels suffer the least. Bone-density loss could be predicted by declining levels of DHEA.[5] Dr Alan Gaby, who has worked extensively with DHEA, suggests that it might augment the bone-building effects of progesterone and says that it is the only hormone which appears to be capable of both inhibiting bone reabsorption and stimulating new bone formation.[5] DHEA analogue is available as Youthinol, extracted from Mexican Yam as dioscorea. The initial dosage to stabilise DHEA levels is followed by a lower maintenance dosage.

DHEA should be used under guidance.

▶ *Fluoride*

Fluoride may be prescribed to increase bone formation. However, there is evidence that the new bone is brittle and prone to fracture at the hip — a 3% higher incidence in women.[7] (Fractures of the hip are significantly higher in areas where the water is naturally high in fluoride.) This leads one to wonder what effect fluoridation of water is having on the incidence of osteoporosis. Fluoride toxicity also causes up to 40% of patients to discontinue treatment due to gastrointestinal inflammation, ulcers, bleeding and pain.

▶ *Calcitonin*

Calcitonin is a thyroid hormone which contributes to bone formation. As levels of calcitonin can decrease with age, injections of it have been given to prevent osteoporosis. The body rejects the calcitonin after a period of twelve to eighteen months, so the treatment is short-term.

▶ *Sodium etidronate*

This is used for treating established spinal osteoporosis on a short-term basis. It can adversely affect mineralisation of bone, and increase pain and the risk of non-spinal fractures if taken in high dose or over a long period of time.

▶ *Alendronate* (Fosamax)

The manufacturers of the anti-osteoporosis drug Alendronate have now admitted that it causes severe side-effects[8] including ulceration of the oesophagus.

▶ *Chinese herbs for osteoporosis*

Chinese herbs are an extremely effective means of preventing and treating osteoporosis. They have been used for thousands of years and, when properly prescribed, do not have side-effects. Best prescribed by a practitioner of Chinese medicine, they may be combined with other herbs to suit individual needs.

▶ **He Shou Wu** *(Polygonium multifolium or Chinese Cornbind)*

A tonic herb, He Shou Wu is taken over an extended period of time and may be combined with a yin tonic such as *Rehmannia glutinosa*. It appears to actually reverse osteoporosis. He Shou Wu also lowers blood cholesterol levels. The herb is usually taken for three months and then repeated as often as necessary after a break of two or three months. The recommended dose is one dessertspoon of the tincture daily. It is also available as a powder or tablets.

▶ **Siberian Ginseng** *(Eleutherococcus)*

In addition to treating and preventing osteoporosis, Siberian Ginseng has an anti-rheumatic action and anti-stress and anti-fatigue properties, so is an ideal herb for menopause. (It should not be confused with other forms of ginseng.) It can also normalise blood sugar levels and stimulate the immune system.

▶ **Homoeopathy**

Homoeopathic medicines are dilute preparations of substances which would cause the same symptoms if they were taken in their usual form. The dilute form contains no molecules of the substances but retains an energetic impression. They are extremely useful when there are contraindications to medical drugs or herbs. Whilst some homoeopathic remedies can be taken as 'first aid' measures, it is sensible to consult a homoeopathic practitioner who will take many factors into account when prescribing for you.

▶ **Sepia**

Where it fits the constitutional picture, Sepia may well help with osteoporosis and osteoarthritis. A 'Sepia patient' is typically dejected, under a gloomy black cloud, and wishes to escape from family commitments. Sepia patients tend to perspire easily. They feel better after exercise and are often fond of dancing.

► **Orachel**

Orachel is a mineral and vitamin formulation which, it is claimed, removes calcium from the plaque deposits in the arteries and relays them to the bone tissue.

References:

1   *WDDTY* Vol. 6 No. 12 p. 1

2   *Cur Res in Osteo and Bone Mine Meas II,* British Institute of Radiology, London, 1992, quoted in *WDDTY* Vol. 6 No. 12

3   *Corticosteroids and Bone,* The National Osteoporosis Society, England, 1996

4   *Osteoporosis reversal with transdermal progesterone,* Lancet 336, 24 November 1990

5   *Bio/Tech News: The Hormone of Life* quotes *Journal of Steroid Biochemistry and Molecular Biology,* 1991, and Interdisciplinary Group on Osteoporosis, Free University of Brussels, Belgium, 1990

6   *Preventing and Reversing Osteoporosis,* AR Gaby, MD, Prima Publishing, 1993

7   *Journal of the American Medical Association,*12 August 1992, quoted in *Natural Progesterone: the multiple role of a remarkable hormone,* John R Lee MD. BLL Publishing, California, 1993

8   *WDDTY* Vol. 7 No. 3
    Corticosteroids and Bone, The Osteoporosis Society, op. cit.

See also:

Menopause Matters, Judy Hall and Dr Robert Jacobs. Element Books, Shaftesbury, England, 1994

Passage to Power, Leslie Kenton. Vermillion, London, 1996

A Book About Menopause, Montreal Health Press Inc.

WDDTY Vol. 3 No. 9; Vol. 6 No. 8 p. 10, No. 7 p. 9, No. 6 p. 1

► *ToDo*

Are you at risk?

Tick the box if any of the following apply to you:

Family history of osteoporosis ☐

Low calcium intake especially in youth ☑

Low body weight ☐

Low bone density ☑

Previous fracture ☐

History of dieting, especially crash type ☑

Anorexia or bulimia nervosa ☐

Lack of appropriate exercise ☑

Early menopause ☑

Of European descent ☑

Have had no children ☐

History of scanty or missing periods ☐

High alcohol intake ☐

High caffeine intake ☐

Excessive intake of cola drinks ☐

History of excessive exercise or training ☐

Inflammatory bowel disease ☐

Rheumatoid arthritis ? ☐

Thyroid disease ☐

Chronic liver and kidney disease ☐

Use of oral corticosteroids (steroid tablets) ☐

Use of diuretics ☐

Heavy smoker ☐

Junk food or high protein diet ☑

High antacid consumption (when containing aluminium) ☐

Oestrogen dominant ☐

Even one tick may mean that you are at risk. It is worth taking preventive measures and adjusting your lifestyle now.

▶ **Check your height**

Ask your partner or a friend to mark your height against a door jamb at three-month intervals. A height loss of 3 mm or more per year can indicate osteoporosis.

▶ **Family history**

Talk to the older female members of your family. Specifically ask them if they appear to have decreased in height over the years. Did their mother or her mother suffer in this way? Did they have spontaneous fractures of wrist, hip, spine or other bones? Did they suffer from low back pain and neck ache? If so, you have a family history of osteoporosis and should take appropriate preventive measures for yourself (and your daughters if you have any).

Take out your old photograph albums. Look at family photos, especially of a couple you can track over the years. Look at your grandparents' wedding photographs and then look at them together in old age. Notice their height in relationship to each other. Does it change? Look at your parents' wedding photographs and then look at them as they grow older. Look at any other couples where the woman is related to you. Pay special attention to the females in your family but remember that osteoporosis affects men as well as women. Compare height over the years. Do the women appear to be shrinking? To be developing dowager's humps? To have lost their necks? Are they still standing tall as they move into their sixties and seventies? Or do they gradually shrink into themselves, bellies extending forward as the spine bows into an 'S' shape, head sinking into the neck and pushing forward onto the chest?

If so, it looks as though you have a family history of osteoporosis and it would be worth consulting a practitioner of Chinese herbalism with a view to taking a herb such as He Shou Wu. Alternatively, consult a Western herbalist regarding natural progesterone.

▶ **Exercise**

What kind of exercise do you do? (Walking the dog counts.)

How long do you exercise for?

How often?

Is it weight-bearing?

Does it put tension on your muscles?

If you lead a sedentary lifestyle, then you should seriously think about taking more exercise. This does not have to be a chore. You don't have to go out jogging or take up aerobics. Simply leaving the car at home, walking briskly to the shops and then carrying the shopping home will dramatically improve your chances of reaching old age without osteoporosis. You could buy some weights and work with them. Or you could enrol at the health club or the gym as some of the exercise should put your muscles under tension. You could get out your bicycle. Twenty minutes of dancing around the living room to some of your old records is equally effective. But you could think about taking up tap or line dancing instead. Going to a yoga, tai chi chuan or qi qong class or some other form of communal exercise is an opportunity to meet new people as well as being an enjoyable form of movement.

Think back to your teens and twenties. What forms of exercise did you enjoy? Can you take any of these up again?

Make a resolution to start now. Search out a suitable class or get walking!

▶ *Diet*

As more than two cups of coffee or three of tea per day can exacerbate osteoporosis, and eating well can greatly improve it, it makes sense to adjust your diet (see Diet, page 133).

Heart Disease

Heart disease is not a disease of menopause. However, prior to menopause women have a much lower incidence of heart disease than men. After menopause the incidence of heart disease in women rises to the same level as men. This is believed to reflect the fact that post-menopausal women have higher levels of cholesterol and the blood fats associated with coronary artery disease (low-density lipoproteins). Although the exact reasons for this are unclear, it has been theorised that oestrogens have a protective function prior to menopause. However, it is known that the contraceptive pill, which contains oestrogen, increases the risk of heart and cardiovascular disease because it encourages blood clotting. It also encourages the retention of fluids and salt which can lead to high blood pressure, which in turn increases the likelihood of heart attack, embolism, thrombosis and stroke. The theory that oestrogen could prevent heart attacks was based on the observation that it decreased cholesterol. The body utilises cholesterol to make sex hormones prior to menopause. After menopause, there may be an excess of cholesterol as the body uses less of it for hormone production. (For this reason a high reading of cholesterol may be normal around the end of menopause and it may not be necessary to undertake the drastic cholesterol-lowering diets and drugs often recommended to women at this stage.)

Medical opinion on cholesterol is changing: it is now recognised that there is 'good' cholesterol and 'bad' cholesterol. Cholesterol is the base substance, the building block, from which the body makes all its steroid hormones — essential for efficient functioning of body processes. Lack of the 'right' kind of cholesterol can therefore be as detrimental to health as a surfeit of the 'wrong' kind. There is a proven link between low cholesterol, especially naturally low levels, and suicide.[1]

▶ *FactFile*

▶ *Vitamin E*

Vitamin E in a dose of 100 mg daily has been shown to reduce heart and circulatory disease in women by 46% percent.[2] It also has a beneficial effect on several menopausal problems. Vitamin E is best taken with vitamin C and selenium which aid absorption. Women with high blood pressure, diabetes and existing heart trouble should only take vitamin E under the supervision of a nutritional specialist as it can exacerbate the condition. The situation with women who have medical conditions precluding oestrogen (cancer of the breast and uterus, fibroids, endometriosis) is unclear. Studies had indicated avoiding added vitamin E as it may raise oestrogen levels, but a French study showed that mean vitamin E levels were significantly lower in breast cancer patients than in controls[3] and that this might be associated with a low antioxidant status. It has been suggested that the raised oestrogen levels may be associated with natural oestrogens present in the refined soy oil used in some vitamin E preparations.[4] The best way to take vitamin E is in unprocessed foodstuffs.

Vitamin E rich foods include: cold pressed oils such as sunflower and safflower, eggs, wheatgerm, organ meats, whole grains, avocados, nuts (especially hazelnuts), tomatoes, cucumbers, dark green leafy vegetables, brown rice and seeds.

▶ *Selenium*

Selenium deficiency has been linked to increased risk of furred-up arteries. Selenium occurs naturally in the soil and is found in cereals, bread, meat and poultry. However, British soils are deficient in selenium so supplementation may be required. The best way to take additional selenium is through diet as it is toxic in relatively low doses (600 mg per day). Supplementation through the mineral should be limited to 50-200 mg daily.

Dietary sources of selenium: brazil nuts, tuna, onions, tomatoes and broccoli.

▶ *Fruit*

Studies have shown that healthy eaters consuming four pieces of fresh fruit every day have a 24% reduction in fatal heart disease, a 32% reduction in death from stroke, and an overall 21% lower mortality rate. Vegetarians have a 15% lower rate of fatal heart disease, those who eat wholemeal bread every day a 12% reduction, and those who have a raw salad every day a 26% lower rate.[5] Dried figs contain pectin, a soluble fibre which is believed to lower cholesterol.

▶ *Exercise*

Exercise has a beneficial effect in preventing heart disease. It has to be aerobic exercise (creating sustained raised heart rate) over a period of thirty minutes, three times a week. A brisk walk, swimming, cycling, running, dancing and tai chi chuan can all be aerobic.

▶ *Omega-3*

Omega-3 fatty acids (found in fatty fish, soya, sesame seeds, flaxseed) have been shown to decrease the incidence of heart disease dramatically. Choose fish oils with a high Omega-3 content. If you are a vegetarian, the linoleic acid found in leafy green vegetables also protects you. Whether you are a vegetarian or not, extra fibre is also required to protect your heart.

▶ *HRT and heart disease*

Preventing heart disease is the second most commonly cited reason for prescribing HRT. The evidence is far from clear, however. One study which purported to show that HRT halved the risk of heart disease had such serious flaws that the editorial in the journal in which it was reported criticised it.[6] Further study of previous research has shown that the samples were 'self-selected'. The most likely users of HRT are white, upper middle class, slim, educated and therefore at less risk of heart disease anyway. And in one study it was suggested that the risk of heart disease was actually increased by HRT.[7] (A study on men had to be stopped when the incidence of heart attacks rose sharply.[7]) The studies have been carried out on women who were given oestrogen only. These women were generally healthier and more carefully selected than women given HRT today. It is known that progestogen, now given for part of the cycle to reduce the cancer risk, adversely affects cholesterol.

New studies are under way to evaluate the effects of combined HRT. In the latest, by the Imperial Cancer Research team's unit at Oxford, Sir Richard Doll, a leading cancer epidemiologist, claims that HRT *might* reduce the risk of heart disease by as much as 30%.[8]

▶ *Cholesterol-lowering drugs*

Cholesterol-lowering drugs such as Zocor may be prescribed for high levels of cholesterol. However, there are well documented dangers to the liver, so frequent liver function tests are essential. Patients who are heavy drinkers or who have a history of liver disease are at special risk. In addition, researchers at the University of California claim that these drugs, and in particular fibrates and statins, are cancer-inducing.[9]

▶ ***Natural hormones***

Natural hormones are derived from plants. They have a similar action to the hormones found in the body. (They should not be confused with synthetic hormones which may be made from the same source but have their molecular structure altered.) They combine with the same receptors as the body's own hormones, but may not activate them in the same way. Thus the plant-derived hormones may not have the same risks attached to them as taking synthetic 'human' hormones such as oestrogen and progestogen.

▶ ***DHEA*** *(Dehydroepiandosterone)*

DHEA is a naturally occurring steroid hormone produced in the adrenal glands of the human body. It has been called the 'mother hormone' because the body can convert it into oestrogen and testosterone and, indirectly, into progesterone.[7] Low levels of DHEA have been linked with heart disease in men[10] and Alan R Gaby, MD claims that supplementing with natural DHEA of plant origin has been shown to lower the 'bad' form of cholesterol (LDL) and so may help to prevent heart disease.[11] DHEA analogue dioscorea is extracted from Mexican wild yam and sold as Youthinol and other brand names. The suggested usage is one tablet or more twice daily according to need.

▶ ***Wild yam cream***

The natural progesterone in wild yam cream is claimed to normalise blood clotting and reduce sodium and fluid retention and may therefore prevent embolism, thrombosis and high blood pressure (see Natural HRT).

▶ *Chinese medicine*

The Chinese herb He Shou Wu has the property of lowering cholesterol levels. It should be taken under the supervision of a Chinese medicine practitioner.

▶ *Orachel*

Orachel is a natural oral chelation treatment which appears to remove plaque from arteries without side-effects. It stimulates the secretion of high-density lipoproteins (HDL). HDL prevents cholesterol being deposited in the artery walls. It also dissolves the fat and breaks up the plaque.[11]

▶ *Foliate*

Foliate has a protective function for the lining of the arteries. Recommended dose is 400 mg daily.

References

1   *WDDTY* Vol. 7 No. 8

2   Report on American Heart Association Meeting in New Orleans, *Medical World News,* December 1992, p.,16-17

3   *Int J Cancer* 67(2) 170-75 17 July 1996, quoted in *Positive Health* Issue 17, 1997

4   Jeff Millar in an Internet conversation with Debby Howard

5   *BMJ,* 1996, 313:775-79

6   *New England Journal of Medicine* 15 April 1993

7   *WDDTY* Vol. 6 No. 12 p. 7

8   Quoted in *The Lancet* 10.97, op. cit.

9   *Positive Health Magazine* April/May 1996

10 *Bio/Tech News: The Hormone of Life*

11 *Preventing and Reversing Osteoporosis,* Alan Gaby. Prima Publishing, 1993. Johns Hopkins Department of Medicine Research, 1988
    WDDTY Vol. 4 No. 9 p. 3; Vol. 7 No. 5

12 Tom Mower, President of Neways International Ltd

▶ *ToDo*

▶ *Are you at risk?*

Tick the boxes that apply to you?

Smoker ☐

Overweight ☐

Sedentary lifestyle ☐

High stress level ☐

Poor diet and nutrition ☐

High alcohol intake ☐

High coffee intake ☐

Family history ☐

High blood fats ☐

If you made one tick or more: consider adjusting your lifestyle

▶ *Steps to reduce heart disease*

Stop smoking

Maintain a normal body weight

Eat a diet high in natural fibre and low in animal fats (the role of which is currently being reassessed so this advice might change)

Switch to fish oils and cook with olive oil

Eat plenty of fresh fruit and a walnut a day

Avoid caffeinated coffee, tea and soft drinks

Exercise appropriately

Reduce stress

▶ *Check out your family history*

Check with older members of your family the incidence of heart and cardiovascular disease within the family.

▶ *Change your lifestyle*

Exercise is one of the most important preventive steps. Ensure that you exercise at least three times a week for thirty minutes. A brisk walk would do.

Reduce your stress. Learn to recognise your stress triggers (the menopause diary is helpful here).

Note down the situations that make you feel wound up, tense, anxious, put you under pressure:

Is there a way to offload some of these? e.g. renegotiate your work load, rearrange your hours, job share, etc.

How much time do you take each day for yourself?

What nourishes you, revitalises you? What makes you feel good?

How long do you spend on this?

Can you make more time?

How?

If you have a job and a house to maintain, you may need to think about getting in a cleaner. You may need to look at sharing jobs around the house, or the office. Bringing in a friend might produce an answer. Discuss with her all your options. Often an outsider's view shows us something we have missed.

▶ *Exercise*

The exercise needed to prevent heart disease is aerobic — that is, it makes you breathless and needs sustained work. It also needs to be something that you can keep up. It is no good going running for a couple of weeks and then losing interest. Enrolling at your local health club or leisure centre would be a good start. Getting together with a group of friends also encourages you to be regular in your exercise. A class for which you have paid in advance is likely to make you more committed and it may well be more fun to exercise with other people. But exercise can be simple. Walking or cycling to the shops, to work or to the train each day could give you all the exercise you need. If you travel by bus or tube, getting on a couple of stops from home could be enough to make a difference. Walk in the park at lunchtime. Go out for a morning run. Or join a class for tai chi chuan or aerobics. You will not only feel better but you will sleep better too, as healthy exercise promotes sleep.

What kind of exercise can you sustain an interest in?

Do you have friends who would join you?

What could you do each day to make a difference?

Check with your local library about what kind of exercise classes are available.

Start right now!

▶ *Learn to relax*

Relax for at least 20 minutes each day, more if possible. Two sessions per day are ideal. (If you travel to work on public transport, you can adapt this exercise slightly, tape it on a walkman, and do it on the way to and from work).

Basic relaxation

Ensure that you will not be disturbed for the length of time you wish to relax. If you are constrained by time and will worry about how much time has passed, use a timer to indicate when the period has elapsed. However, the timer should have a quiet tone; being roughly jolted out of relaxation is uncomfortable and counter-productive. Suitable music helps with relaxation and can be used to time the session. Sit or lie comfortably, preferably in loose clothing. The exercise can either be taped, leaving pauses where appropriate, or memorised (it can be helpful to have a friend read it to you for the first few sessions):

Have your eyes open to begin with, slowly closing and opening them on each number as you count backwards from ten to one. This will relax your eyelids and, when you have finished the count, you can close your eyes and leave them closed until the end of the session.

Notice how relaxed your eyelids feel, how they lie softly against the bottom lid. Then allow this feeling of relaxation to spread across your forehead and face. If you are aware of any tension, screw up your face and then let it relax. If your scalp feels tight, raise and lower your eyebrows to release the tension.

Allow the feeling of relaxation to flow down into your neck and shoulders. If your shoulders feel tight, contract, raise and lower them and let go to release the tension.

Be aware of your arms as the waves of relaxation move down them. Clench and unclench your fists to release the tension, then allow the relaxation to move right down into your finger tips until your arms lie loose beside you.

Allow the feeling of relaxation to flow down into your chest, taking a few deep, slow breaths and breathing out any tension you may be aware of. Then allow the feeling of peace and relaxation to move down into your diaphragm, sensing it soften and relax as you breathe.

Move your breath down into your belly and breathe out any tension you may feel there. Your belly should be relaxed; let it hang out.

Be aware of your hips and lower back and allow the relaxation to flow through them. If there is any tension, contract the buttocks and then let go.

Allow the waves of relaxation to move down into your legs and feet. To free any tension, pull the knees downwards to tighten and contract, and then release. Pull the feet up and then relax. The sense of peace and relaxation should then flow right down to your toes.

Now check that your whole body is feeling loose and relaxed.

Allow your breathing to slow still further, letting the abdominal muscles do the breathing for you and taking a pause between each in and out breath. Let yourself be still for a few minutes, enjoying this sense of total relaxation and peace.

▶ (If you wish to do a short relaxation, the session can terminate here — in which case move to the final instructions **)

As you continue to breathe in a sense of peace and relaxation, become aware that you are surrounded by light. Breathe this light into your heart, feeling it fill and become energised.

When your heart is full of light, let it spill out and flow up to your head and down to your feet. Continue gently to breathe in more and more light and let it flow through your body, washing away any pain, stiffness or worries. When you are completely full of light, simply relax and enjoy the sensation of absolute peace.

***When you are ready to end the session, begin to breathe a little deeper and become aware of the weight of your body once more. Draw the light around you to cocoon yourself like an egg. Your body will remain relaxed and free from tension. Slowly count from one to ten, by which time you will be wide awake and very alert. Open your eyes and return your attention to the room.*

▶ (Note: If you wish to fall asleep after this exercise, simply omit the final instructions ** and substitute the following *)

**Continue to breathe rhythmically, allowing your breathing to deepen until you drift gently into sleep. You will sleep for as long as you wish, waking refreshed and full of vitality.*

Diet and Nutrition

What you put into your body affects your health

A good, balanced diet is essential at any time of life but it can make all the difference at menopause.

The ideal diet is a varied wholefood one, containing as little processed food as possible, and including a high proportion of fresh vegetables and fruits providing trace elements and vitamins. Ideally these should be organic to avoid pesticides and other toxins. Include sprouted seeds, beans and grains. As too much protein can affect calcium take-up, red meat should be limited. Try to avoid excessive consumption of tea and coffee — herbal teas and mineral water help to cleanse the body.

Soya beans, sweetcorn, maize, tomatoes and other vegetables are now being genetically engineered (and may still be sold as 'organic'). They may contain genetic pesticides, 'natural' antibiotics and other unwholesome substances. They will obviously be detrimental to health, as will food that has been irradiated to keep longer. Check before you buy.

Some body types cannot take raw food. If you suffer from bloating and flatulence, try cooking your vegetables and avoid raw salads.

Many of the menopausal problems women encounter can be food-allergy-based. If you suspect food allergies might be present, or if you have problems with obesity or toxicity and tiredness, try the detox diet. Food should be organic wherever possible.

Avoiding a food you are allergic to for six months is often enough to remove the allergy.

Avoid additives and preservatives where possible — they add to your toxic load.

▶ *FactFile*

▶ **Sources of vitamin E**

Cold pressed oils: sunflower, safflower • Eggs • Wheatgerm
Organ meats • Whole grains • Wholemeal bread • Avocado
Nuts • Tomatoes • Cucumbers • Leafy vegetables

▶ **Sources of vitamin C**

Citrus fruits • Rosehips • Strawberries • Broccoli • Tomatoes
Peppers

▶ **Sources of selenium**

Meats • Dairy products • Brewers yeast • Fish • Grains

▶ **Sources of Vitamin B$_6$**

Whole grains • Milk • Yeast • Egg yolk • Brown rice • Bran

The detox diet

Breakfast: Cooked, pre-soaked dried fruit including apricots, peaches, pears, figs, prunes, apples (note: cooked fresh apples can be included).

Lunch: Home-made vegetable soup, miso soup or steamed vegetables with brown rice.

Supper: Brown rice with steamed vegetables or, occasionally, stir-fried in virgin olive oil.

Drink: Drink as little as possible. Mineral water or herb teas only. No tea, coffee or alcohol.

Do not use: Anything you are allergic to. Avoid: Sugar, salt, bread, dairy foods, tomatoes, citrus fruit, raw foods — fruit should be cooked.

Note: *Use as wide a variety of vegetables as possible, including sea vegetables and sprouted legumes and grains. Brown rice can be cooked with garlic and a little fresh ginger. Herbs can be added to soups and vegetables for flavouring. Tahini paste (rich in calcium) can be thinned with water to make a sauce for occasional use.*

Follow the strict diet for 2-4 weeks, then gradually introduce non-allergenic foods again, stopping immediately if an adverse effect is noticed. Symptoms may get worse before they get better as the detoxifying process gets under way, but within two weeks the condition should have improved dramatically. An added benefit can be a weight loss of about 7 lbs in the first week or two without any hunger pangs.

A juice fast can also be highly beneficial if your body can stand it (some people find fasting makes them too lightheaded— it depends on body type). If possible, use fresh organic fruits and vegetables for juicing at home (juicers are readily available). Otherwise, buy organic juices from the health food store. Include leafy green vegetables (but avoid too much spinach as it contains oxalic acid). Try some of the less obvious combinations: beetroot, carrot and orange is highly sustaining. Whilst on the juice fast, drink plenty of mineral water. You can include herb teas but no tea, coffee or other beverages and no alcohol.

▶ *ToDo*

Become much more aware of what you eat. Keep a detailed food diary for a week or two. Note down every single thing that passes your lips. Note especially the things you crave—these may indicate food allergy but can also be a symptom of a trace element mineral shortage as, left to itself, your body knows what you need to eat. Note all the drinks you take, even water. At the end of each day, add them up. You may be surprised how many cups of coffee or tea you drink in a day.

Do you recognise or suspect any food allergies?

Have you noticed a correlation between a particular food and a set of symptoms? If you suspect food allergy, try the detox diet and then gradually restart foods. Stop immediately if symptoms recur.

Adjust your diet to include as much fresh wholefood as possible.

For maximum energy, and PMS reduction, try a sustained-release diet with a high-fibre carbohydrate base such as brown rice or other cooked grain, wholemeal bread and wholewheat pasta eaten at frequent intervals (five meals per day instead of three).

Avoid sugar as much as possible as an underlying blood sugar disorder may create menopausal 'symptoms'.

Tick the box if any of the following apply to you:

Low blood sugar ☐

Do you frequently feel faint and dizzy? ☐

Do you break out in cold sweats? ☐

Does your energy level fluctuate suddenly? ☐

Do you have feelings of panic and disorientation? ☐

Do you feel irritable if you don't eat? ☐

Do you crave sweets and sugary foods? ☐

Do you feel worse 1-2 hours later? ☐

If you have ticked three or more of the above, there is a possibility you may have low blood sugar. This cannot be diagnosed on a straightforward single blood sugar measurement but needs a special test called a Six-Hour Glucose Tolerance test, which any doctor or hospital can perform.

Treatment: Treatment should include a high-fibre diet and avoidance of refined and added sugar. Supplements which contain chromium, such as brewers yeast, may help (but avoid brewers yeast if you suffer from candida). A naturopathic, homoeopathic or herbal practitioner should be able to help. Apart from dietary advice, there is nothing that conventional medicine can offer for this condition.

Peach-Flowered Tea-Tree (Bush) helps to stabilise blood sugar levels.

Use as much 'green energy' as possible — including sea vegetables (available from health food stores, some supermarkets and Chinese stores).

Avoid crash dieting. The detox diet will help you to lose weight if you feel this is essential.

Change to naturally decaffeinated coffee (some decaffeinated coffees use chemicals) and organic tea, preferably decaffeinated. Where possible limit your consumption of tea and coffee. Replace with herb teas, fruit juices and mineral water.

Start reading the labels on foods! Many contain hidden sugar and high salt and some products sold in Britain contain artificial sweeteners that are banned in the United States because of their carcinogenic properties. Many foods also contain soya, so you may unwittingly be consuming genetically altered beans.

▶ *Jottings*

IV: Mood

Change is mourning for things ended
Regret for things undone now never to be known

Mood

Emotions and feelings play an important part in midlife change. Fluctuating moods, anxiety and depression are associated by the medical profession with menopause. They are put down to 'your hormones'. It is true that hormones do play a role. When your hormonal balance is out of kilter, you are too. Even if you are normally the most contented and happy of women, you might notice that you are weepy or irritable from time to time. You may also be aware of moments of extreme elation, a sudden joy that rises up out of nowhere. Perhaps you have put it down to your age — most women do. It happens to almost all menopausal women at one time or another. It is part of 'The Change' and may well indicate nothing more than a hormone surge. However, there may be something much deeper going on below the irrational, superficial mood swings.

How do you feel?

How you feel is an indication of how you are — on all levels. It sounds simple, and yet most people don't realise this, or if they do they don't acknowledge it. Feelings and emotions are not good or bad, they just are. But you might have been taught that it is 'not nice' to feel anger, sadness or even great joy. On the whole, people do not fully express what they are feeling. They hold back, suppress. Sometimes this process has become so automatic that they do not know they are feeling anything at all. When asked how they are, they reply, 'Fine,' regardless of whether it is true or not. Or they launch into a long list of symptoms that still does not answer the question: 'How are *you?*' 'You' is not just a body. 'You' is a person. A person with feelings. You can be feeling fine and still be experiencing symptoms. Or you can have no symptoms at all, and be feeling absolutely awful. You feel feelings, you have symptoms.

How often do you stop to ask yourself, 'Am I really fine?' If you did, you might well say: 'Well, yes, I've got a headache but apart from that I feel fine,' and this will be true. On a feeling level you really are OK. On the other hand, you might say: 'I know I've got a headache and I shouted at the kids this morning, and then I cried a bit, but I really am fine, aren't I?' If you sit down and *think* about it further, then you may say: 'Well, yes, I know I'm under a bit of pressure at the moment. My eldest daughter is just off to university and I've got a lot to do to get her ready. I'll miss her. So maybe deep down I'm not quite so fine as I thought I was.' If you sit down and let yourself *feel* it, you may well burst into tears. Or you may even come out in a hot sweat or some other 'menopausal symptom'. So, in this case, you are not fine on a feeling level, and that may well have a great deal to do with the symptoms you have had.

▶ *ToDo*

So, how are you? How do you feel? Write down what is going on in your life, and how you feel about it. Don't worry if those feelings are happy, sad, irrational, senseless, 'good', 'bad'. Just let it pour onto the paper.

Take the time to honour and acknowledge those feelings. To say: 'Yes, this is how I feel.' Don't judge those feelings, just allow them to be.

Then take a look through your menopause diary. What feelings are you recording under Mood? What is your most frequent emotion? Is there an underlying theme? Have you already noticed a link between life-events and the feelings you are experiencing?

Go back to the life statement you made when you started this book. Did you say: 'I am a women who feels . . .'? Is there anything you want to add to it?

Before we look more deeply into how you are feeling, we need to establish whether you are simply going through the normal emotional ups and downs of midlife or whether there is a more serious mood disturbance going on. If you know you really are fine, then skip the next section. But if you have suffered from ongoing depression, panic or anxiety, or are experiencing mood disturbances, then it may help you.

Anxiety and Depression

While most women will only suffer a few mood swings, anxiety and depression may nevertheless accompany the menopause and quite commonly precede it by a year or two. The good news is that incidence of depression drops sharply one year after menopause. So, even if you have suffered depression prior to and during the menopause, you are unlikely to do so afterwards. Anxiety and panic attacks may be part of depression, but they can have other causes.

Depression is often treated with antidepressants and addictive tranquillisers, sleeping pills, beta-blockers or HRT. Endogenous depression does appear to benefit from antidepressants; they can stabilise the underlying chemical imbalance. Reactive depression, anxiety and panic attacks, on the other hand, benefit from counselling and psychotherapy. Antidepressants have little effect. Natural remedies can have a profoundly beneficial effect on both types of depression.

▶ *FactFile*

There is a statistical increase in depression amongst women aged between 45 and 49. This continues for one year after menopause and then drops sharply.

Depression improves dramatically after menopause.

Two types of depression:

Endogenous: Appears to have a biochemical basis, and can be linked to changing hormone levels. May be helped by antidepressants, acupuncture or natural remedies.

Reactive: Linked to life-events and stress. May be helped by counselling and stress-reduction techniques. Unlikely to respond to antidepressants.

▶ **Panic attacks:**

First aid: Five deep, slow breaths. If breathing is fast and shallow or gasping, put a large paper bag over head (to remedy over-breathing) or cup hands around nose. Take **Rescue Remedy.** Inhale lavender oil — a few drops on a handkerchief will last all day.

May be helped by tranquillisers or herbal remedies. There may an underlying reason for a panic attack, including low blood sugar. Counselling or psychotherapy may help.

Some medically prescribed drugs can cause depression, as may some synthetically perfumed air-fresheners and other products.[1]

▶ **ToDo**

If you are suffering from depression, then finding out which kind can help you to choose the appropriate treatment:

	yes	no
Do you suffer from disturbed sleep and insomnia?	☐	
Have you lost your appetite?	☐	
Do you wake up early?	☐	
Do you feel terrible at the beginning of the day?	☐	
Do you feel useless, unwanted, rejected, miserable?	☐	
Do happy events make you feel better?	☐	☐
Do stressful events make you feel worse?	☐	☐
Do you feel better talking things over with someone?	☐	☐

Do you eat for comfort? ☐

Do you suffer from stress? ☐

Do you sleep well? ☐

Do you wake feeling good, then get worse
as the day progresses? ☐

Do you feel that an event triggered your depression? ☐

If you have ticked the first four or five boxes and answered No to the three Yes/No questions, it is likely that you are suffering from endogenous depression. You may be helped by antidepressants, acupuncture and natural remedies.

If you answered Yes to the three Yes/No questions and ticked the boxes following them, then you are likely to be suffering from reactive depression. You may find that counselling or psychotherapy helps.

▶ ***Do you have panic attacks?***

	yes	no
Do you feel anxious, suffer from sweaty palms, a thumping heart, dizziness, gasp for breath?	☐	☐
Do you find it difficult to be in enclosed spaces or amongst a crowd?	☐	☐
Do you worry a lot?	☐	☐

Strange as it may sound, putting your head in a large paper bag and breathing normally is excellent first aid for panic attacks. When you panic, you tend to hyperventilate and take in too much oxygen. Breathing into a paper bag counteracts this with carbon dioxide.

Rescue Remedy (a Bach Flower Remedy available from many chemists and health food shops) will also help. For longer-term treatment, counselling or psychotherapy could help you to uncover the reasons why you have the attacks. Natural remedies, such as other flower essences and homoeopathy, may also help.

Panic attacks may be indicative of low blood-sugar. A high-fibre diet and supplements containing chromium, such as brewers yeast, can help, as can homoeopathy or herbalism. Apart from advising on diet, there is nothing conventional medicine can do for this condition.

▶ *Breathing*

Chronic anxiety tends to go with fast, shallow breathing.

Place your hands over your solar plexus, fingers touching, and breathe in:

	yes	no
Do your shoulders go up?	☐	☐
Do your fingers part?	☐	☐

If you tick yes for the first and not the second, then you are breathing shallowly. Try breathing to a different pattern:

Breathe in to the count of four. Take the breath right down into your belly — which will push out slightly (you can check this by placing your fingers just below the waist with your fingertips just touching. As you breathe in, they will part). Hold your breath for a count of three. Breathe out for five — your belly will pull back in as the lungs empty. Hold your breath for a count of three. Repeat ten to twenty times. Gradually increase the count as you become more proficient.

Whenever you find yourself in a situation that makes you feel anxious, remember to breathe to this new pattern.

▶ *FactFile*

▶ *Natural treatments for depression*

There are many non-addictive remedies available that can help but which need to be tailored to you. Herbal preparations that contain natural tranquillisers can be obtained from health food shops. Homoeopathy, Chinese medicine, herbalism and acupuncture can all help to correct underlying energy or chemical imbalances.

▶ **St Johns Wort** *(Hypericum perforatum)*

St Johns Wort has been used for centuries to counteract anxiety, depression and nervous tension. Studies have shown that St Johns Wort is at least as effective as antidepressants in treating these conditions and has no side-effects.[1] It can be purchased from health food stores as tablets or drops, or taken as a decoction.

▶ **Acupuncture**

Acupuncture has a naturally calming and relaxing effect. Research has shown that it raises endorphin levels. Endorphins act like natural antidepressants.

▶ **Warratah** *(Bush)*

This Australian Bush Essence is excellent for treating black, suicidal depression. It can be taken every ten minutes in extreme cases and then 7 drops three times a day for a week or so afterwards.

▶ **Mustard** *(Bach)*

Mustard is useful for melancholy, black depression and deep gloom arising out of the blue without known cause.

▶ **Pink Fairy Orchid** *(LE)*

This essence is particularly appropriate when depression and panic attacks are brought on by sensitivity to environmental stress, a stressful work place, and groups of people.

▶ **Pulsatilla**

A constitutional homoeopathic remedy, Pulsatilla helps women who are excessively weepy and in need of consolation. The Pulsatilla patient tends to be emotionally extreme, easily moved to tears and laughter.

Your constitutional remedy, properly prescribed by a homoeopath, may well help you to deal with depression. It tends to gently ease the cause of the problem to the surface.

▶ *For panic attacks:*

Rescue Remedy (Bach) quickly treats any kind of shock or panic

Pink Fairy Orchid (LE)

Chromium (if cause is low blood-sugar)

Acupressure: See page 103 for mind-calming points

▶ *For low blood-sugar:*

Peach-Flowered Tea-Tree (Bush) balances low blood sugar.

Enhancing self-esteem

Depression and anxiety are often accompanied by low self-esteem — a feeling that you are worthless, that nobody wants you, that you just aren't special enough. Even if you are not depressed, this is a feeling that can strike without warning during menopause.

▶ *ToDo*

Buy yourself a large scrap-book. Use this to keep anything that enhances your self-esteem, anything that makes you feel better about yourself. If someone buys you a present, take a photo and stick it in the book. Press a flower and stick it in. Keep cards, labels, letters. If someone says something nice about you, write it in the book. Try to make an entry every day. If no one else says anything, find something good about yourself and write it in. Notice, and record, the good points about your body. Put in all the thoughtful things you do for others, and the skills and talents you show. Put in any photos that make you feel special; you can add in close friends and family — the people who support and value you. Whatever you like. Then, when you are feeling low, look at your book. You are special!

How Do I Feel About Menopause?

Everyone approaches menopause with different and mixed feelings. Some of these will be optimistic: looking forward to fresh possibilities, new freedom, a new lease of life. Others will be pessimistic: looking forward to doom, gloom and going downhill. Because of the contradictory nature of midlife, someone who has been a career woman all her life may suddenly find herself facing a very different side of her nature, one that wants to retire from the world and turn inward. If you are a woman who has invested all of herself in her children, and they are now leaving home, you may find yourself embroiled in the 'empty nest syndrome' with its sense of loss and feelings of grief. On the other hand, you may find yourself with a new sense of freedom. Many different emotions surface at midlife: anger, fear, resentment, bitterness, regret, joy, hope. You will have begun to identify some of these from your menopause diary and the work you have already done in this book.

▶ *ToDo*

Allow yourself twenty to thirty minutes of undisturbed time alone. If necessary, take the phone off the hook. Bring the word 'menopause' into your mind. Then add another word: 'my menopause'. Notice how your body reacts. Do you find yourself going tense? Pulling back a bit? Pushing it away, even? Do you find yourself swallowing hard? What sort of emotions are trying to rise up? Do you catch yourself thinking: 'It couldn't happen to me'? Let whatever feelings are there grow. Don't cut them off, don't censor any spontaneous thoughts, but concentrate on your feelings. Simply start writing and let all your thoughts and feelings connected with menopause flow onto the paper.

If you get stuck, you can turn your attention to some of the following questions:

What do I regret about menopause?

Am I angry about anything?

What will I miss?

What do I look forward to about menopause?

What are the emotions that are surfacing around it?

When you are sure you have explored this thoroughly, take some time to review what you have written. Go over all the things you are looking forward to. See if you can bring some of them into being now. Make a 'Looking Forward To' list of them and stick it where you will see it often. Then look at the regrets and emotions that arise. Are there certain themes that come up? A common one is the 'past my sell-by date' scenario. It has several variations but they all tend to go along the lines of being over the hill, past it, getting too old, becoming useless. Another common theme is: 'Nobody will want me any more.' This one is usually linked to children — or husbands — leaving home; or perhaps to redundancy or looming early retirement. Another theme is: 'It's too late for all the things I dreamed of.' Maybe the theme that is coming up is: 'It's time I took my freedom and did something.' What emotions lie behind these feelings? Some of the feelings may be valid in the present moment, but others may be a carryover from the past. You may be carrying emotional baggage that you didn't even know you had — or maybe you did and just did not know how to let go of it.

Letting go is the key. The emotions and feelings of midlife are real and valid at the time, but if you hold on to them for too long, they fester and create the more destructive emotions of resentment, rage and bitterness. This in turn can become an ingrained attitude to life that really does set the pattern for a downhill slide into old age.

Anger

Anger is not a 'bad' emotion. You may have been taught in childhood that it is, in which case you will find it difficult to allow yourself to feel angry — and that anger may turn round and come at you from a different direction. You may also have learnt in childhood that it was something to be feared, so you bend over backwards not to provoke anger in other people. How many times have you been been angry but not shown it, and then have gone out and banged into something or dropped something? The anger may go underground and then surface explosively in another situation, one where you unconsciously sense it is safer to let it out. You can be made to feel rather stupid by a garage mechanic, for instance, but you don't say anything. Then, when you get home, the dog gets under your feet and you lash out. Expressing the anger when it arose would have been cleaner, and could well have saved you that thumping headache and hot flush.

Anger can be a very positive emotion for change. If you become angry enough about something, and can harness that energy, you can achieve anything you set your mind to. If you become angry and cannot focus the energy, then it festers and eats away at you. Menopause is one of those times in life when repressed feelings come whooshing up to the surface. So, if you have held in your anger over the years, this is when it will reappear. The anger may be new, however. Anger at yourself for 'being incompetent' is quite common when hormonal changes affect your memory and coordination. The events in your life may be making you angry. Unfortunately, midlife is a time when partners may decide to leave and pursue their own dreams of lost youth, teenage children may be particularly obstreperous, and parents may be demanding care. You may be saddled with obligations and burdens you would rather not have. Anger can be a natural consequence of these and many other situations.

If you find you are holding on to anger, you have three choices. You can continue to hold on to it. You can accept that it happened and let it go. Or you can do something to change the situation. One of the examples that comes up at midlife is having had surgery, a hysterectomy for example. Even where it was unavoidable, you may well find that you feel angry about it. If you were treated inconsiderately, or not given enough information or choice, then you will almost certainly be angry. You may have felt frustrated, helpless, invaded, not in control of your body. Whilst you cannot turn back the clock and undo the operation, you can express your feelings about it. You can write to your surgeon. If the surgeon is no longer around, you can still write the letter and then tear it up into little pieces or burn it. You could also resolve to do something to help women in a similar situation. Join a self-help group or volunteer to go into hospital to visit women who are having the same operation. You could also try forgiveness. This is deeply healing for your soul and it enables you to let go.

If your husband has walked out and left you, then you can write to him. It helps if you begin: 'When so and so happened, I was angry. I felt . . .' (Stating how you felt is preferable to piling blame on the other person. Blame puts them on the defensive and they will never understand how you felt — or feel, if you are conveying a present anger.) Here again, if you can forgive, it will enable you to let go and move on.

► *ToDo*

Tick the things that apply to you:

I get angry very easily	☐
I find it hard to show anger	☐
I was never allowed to be angry as a child	☐
I always think what I could have said when it's too late	☐
I get frightened if people are angry	☐
My parents never showed anger	☐
One or both of my parents was always angry	☐
I like to keep the peace at all costs	☐
I brood about situations where I was angry but didn't show it	☐
Deep down inside I'm deeply angry	☐

You might well find some links between your upbringing and your ability to show anger.

Now go over what you have done so far and see if you have an 'angry list'. There may be only one item on it, or you may find several, or even many. Gather them all together and write a statement:

'I am angry about _____ '

Take each one in turn:

Is it something you can let go of? ☐

If not, are you prepared to do something about it? ☐

If you want to do something about it, list the steps you can take and set a date by which you will do it.

Physicalising anger

When you get angry, adrenaline rushes around your body. It is called the 'fight or flight' mechanism. Adrenaline pushes extra energy into your muscles. If you don't do anything with it, the adrenaline remains in your body and causes stress. 'Huffing and puffing', big breaths where you snort and breathe out heavily, can help to dissipate the stress. But even more so, moving around will help to get that adrenaline out of your muscles. Go out for a run. Stomp around. Go out into the garden and slash at the weeds or cut the hedge. Clear out a cupboard. Whatever uses the energy. If you find it difficult to express anger, and especially if you have trouble saying 'No', then you can try the following:

▶ *ToDo*

Find a place where you will not be disturbed — and preferably where you cannot be overheard. Stamp your feet rhythmically, one at a time (you may find it easier to stamp one foot only). You may want to move your arms up and down as well. (Alternatively, bang your fists on a table; pad it with a towel or cushion so you don't hurt yourself.) With each stamp shout 'No' as loud as you can. If you have a picture of the person or the situation in your mind, then direct the 'No' to them but not the anger. Continue as long as possible.

Fear

Midlife is a time when many fears arise. They may be practical: 'How am I going to cope with old age?' Or irrational: 'Nobody is going to want me any more.' Fear may also hold you back from doing what you have always wanted to do: 'I'm not good enough . . .' One of the most important steps you can make in facilitating midlife change is to look at your fears honestly and openly, and then to overcome them.

▶ *ToDo*

Make a list of all the things you are afraid of. Don't worry whether they are rational or irrational, large or small issues. Just write them all down.

Then sort the list out. Look at the major issues first. Have you got practical fears such as 'How will I manage? Will the old age pension be enough to support me/us?' If so, you may need to review your financial arrangements, either alone or with your partner. You may need professional advice. Topping up a pension fund can be done with a lump sum payment, or by instalments. In midlife, insurance is still quite easy to come by, but each year reduces the sum available to you for the same premium. You may find that your children have left home and you now have a house which, to be realistic, is too large for your needs. Selling up could release a cash sum to invest for your old age. You may also need to look at more inventive solutions. If you live alone, could you divide your home up and share with a friend, or let part of it to bring you an income? Could you take in a young person who needs a suitable home (in many areas there are schemes for young people which offer you support and backup). This latter idea might also be the solution if your own children have left home and you feel you are no longer needed.

You might also like to look at doing some training now for something which would be useful and generate an income later. So many women nowadays are training for counselling and complementary therapies that there is a shortage of women offering practical services. Even in counselling training, there are areas that do not attract so many candidates, such as grief and bereavement counselling, for which there is an enormous demand. In the practical area, there is always a need for decorating and soft furnishing but have you thought about carpentry, furniture renovation, plumbing, car maintenance? If you enjoy gardening, there could well be someone who would appreciate help with a garden that is now beyond them. Children need collecting from school, and 'granny-sitting', shopping, ironing and other things need to be done. Many elderly people need help with everyday tasks. The opportunities are endless.

If you are alone and your greatest fear is a lonely old age, then begin now to widen your circle of interests and find new friends. It is a mistake to concentrate all your energy on finding a new partner If this does not work, then you will still be alone, whereas friends and interests will always be there. You may well find that volunteering for a befriending scheme brings a new sense of fulfilment into your life. But there are many other possibilities out there—you just need to put your fear aside and look.

▶ *ToDo*

Go through the whole of your list and see what solutions you can find.

When you come to the irrational fears, you may need to explore these in more depth and find where they are coming from (see Mind, page 182).

Coping with fear

Denying that fear exists does not work. It comes round and trips you up when you least expect it. But acknowledging the fear and then putting it to one side and getting on with things does work. If you find your knees are knocking, then flower essences can help. The original Bach Flower

Essences have several for fear: *Aspen, Cherry Plum, Red Chestnut, Rock Rose* and *Mimulus. Dog Rose* (Bush) helps fears of all kinds and instils confidence.

You can also visualise your fear (See Creative Visualisation, page 188).

▶ *ToDo*

Close your eyes and relax. Let an image come into your mind. Choose an animal to portray your fear. Is it a tiger, wild and untamed? A timid little mouse? Let whatever seems appropriate appear.

Then ask this animal what it needs to make it feel safe. Does it need somewhere secure? Does it need attention? Do you need to pet it and reassure it from time to time? Whatever it needs, promise to supply it (and remember to give attention to this from time to time).

Then let the image gently fade away.

You may like to make this image concrete. Buy yourself a stuffed toy animal. Pet it, talk to it, and let it look after your fear for you.

Loss and grief

As menopause is a time of endings, of letting things go, grief may well accompany this transition. It is also a time when unresolved issues come to the surface once again, so old loss may also bring its share of sadness.

You will already have identified some of your regrets around menopause. When you have read through these again, and worked with them as appropriate, you may like to perform a ritual whereby you burn the list and let your regrets dissolve with the smoke.

You might have identified the loss of your fertility as something that is causing you pain—particularly if you have always wanted to have children but have been unable to. Menopause is a time when you shift away from biological creativity into a different way of generating new life. If you have always lacked a creative outlet, or seen yourself primarily as a mother, then it can be difficult to tune in to this new mode of expressing yourself. Paint, dance, music, movement, words and songs are just some of the ways you can be creative. You might like to begin by finding a means of expressing your grief at the loss of your fertility. Create a mourning ritual, light a candle, plant a tree.

If you have identified specific losses, of a partner, parents, children or anything else, it can be helpful — once you have completed your natural mourning process, including expressing anger if appropriate, and letting go — to change how you perceive this loss. Whilst benefit may not be immediately apparent, loss does open the way for change and it is possible to identify the benefit behind the loss. You might find, for instance, that the death of a much-loved parent has actually opened the way for you to have your own opinions and a very different lifestyle from the one your parent wanted for you. You may find that loss and grief have taught you empathy and caring, and you may want to share that with other people who are going through the same difficulties.

▶ *ToDo*

Describe as fully as possible the loss that you have been through. Explore your feelings in relation to this loss.

Have you completed the mourning process and let go? If not, try **Ignatia 200c** or **Sturt Desert Pea** (Bush).

Look at how that loss has changed your life, or changed you inwardly. Find the benefit behind the loss. Look for possible ways of sharing that benefit with others.

You may find that you need to talk things over with a counsellor from an appropriate organisation who knows about your particular type of loss. If you need immediate help, then do not hesitate to phone the Samaritans.

If you have not completed your mourning, then give yourself 15 minutes or so a day in which to grieve and to feel fully all the emotions that are arising. It doesn't sound long, but if you are deeply experiencing the feelings, it will be enough time. Honour that this is how you feel about that loss. Then let the feelings go and get on with your life for the rest of the day.

Once you have overcome this loss, you may find it beneficial to offer your experience-based services to an appropriate counselling or self-help group.

Empty nest syndrome

Menopause happens to be a time when children leave home. You may still identify strongly with the role of mother. Your children may physically have left home some time ago but in your eyes they may still remain 'children'. If you have been grieving over their leaving, you may well be suffering from 'empty nest syndrome'.

▶ *ToDo*

Tick the boxes that apply to you:

Have your children left home? ☐

Do you miss them dreadfully? ☐

Are you having trouble letting them go? ☐

Do the house and your days feel empty without them? ☐

Do you constantly feel there is something missing? ☐

Do you feel resentful if your children don't phone? ☐

Do you still do your children's washing? ☐

Do you keep your children's rooms as they left them? ☐

Do you feel depressed, weepy, without a focus? ☐

Have you lost your purpose in life? ☐

Do you feel that your useful life has ended? ☐

In a society which tends to value women for their role as mother, it can be devastating for a woman who has seen herself purely in those terms to 'lose' her children. If you are having difficulty in letting them go, and in finding a new role for yourself, then a visualisation may help (taking the Bach Flower Remedy *Walnut* aids this process):

Close your eyes and relax. Breathe gently and let yourself settle down quietly.

Now, picture your child in front of you. Allow that child to be the age they are now, a young (or not so young) adult. Acknowledge that they have now grown up and are ready to leave your care.

See the ties that hold you to that child as 'apron strings' going from you and attaching to your child. Taking a big pair of golden scissors, cut these apron strings. Then, using a healing light, dissolve the ties both from yourself and from your child. See the places where they were attached being healed. Check that there are no hidden apron strings around the back. If there are, then cut and dissolve these too.

When you are sure you have cut all the apron strings, look at your grown-up child with new eyes. Accept that in front of you is an independent person, an individual. Someone for whom you did your best but must now let go so that they can make a life of their own. Resolve to let your child live his or her life not as you see fit but as they do. Support them with love, but do not seek to control. Let unconditional love flow between you. Wish them well in their life. Then picture them wrapped in light, and let them go to their own space — picture them in their world, not yours. See yourself surrounded by light, light that brings you healing and love.

Then slowly bring your attention back into the room, keeping the light around you.

Letting go of the apron strings does not cut off love. Indeed, it shows great love. But it does cut off all the 'oughts, buts and shoulds' that tend to attach to parent-child relationships, and to so-called 'love'. If you have had a difficult relationship with your child, then this visualisation can improve things. You may want to follow it up with a letter telling them that, while you will always love them, you acknowledge them as an adult who is capable of running his or her life and that you will no longer interfere in that life.

Dissolving resentment

Resentment is another emotion that can surface at menopause. Resentment is anger that has festered and gone stale. It lies below the surface and bursts out from time to time. Much of the resentment will no longer have any cause, but it can take all the joy out of life. If you have identified resentment, then you have two choices. To hold on to it and let it spoil your life. Or to let it go and find joy instead.

► *ToDo*

Close your eyes and relax. Think about the things on your list that made you resentful. Take your attention around your body and notice where the resentment is. Check out your abdomen, your womb, your shoulders, your solar plexus. Picture the resentment as 'black energy'.

Now picture a purple crystal just in front of you. This crystal is magnetically charged and can pull the resentment out of your body. Watch as all the black energy is drawn out. Feel it leave your body and see it disappear into the crystal.

When all the black energy has gone into the crystal to be transformed, the crystal will change to a pink one. From the pink crystal will come a stream of pink energy. This will flow into all the places where you were holding the resentment. It will heal those places. Then the stream of pink energy will flow into your heart, filling it up with peace and joy until it is overflowing.

When you have finished the visualisation, open your eyes and feel yourself still surrounded by the pink energy. It will protect and energise you.

Acceptance

There will no doubt be things that have arisen that you would very much like to change, but cannot do so. On the other hand, there will be things that have changed that you wanted to stay the same. Here again you have a choice. You can either accept things as they are, or you can endlessly go over and over the same old ground. There are women who become 'stuck in menopause', to which HRT can be a contributory factor. They do not take the final step that would allow them to move into a new way of being. The key to making this move is acceptance. Acceptance of the past, letting it go. Acceptance of the present moment, living it fully. Acceptance of The Change you are undergoing. And acceptance of the unshaped future to come, allowing it to be, without worrying about what it will be. If you can develop acceptance and embrace change willingly, then you can move on.

You will find positive affirmations helpful here. Affirmations 're-program' you. A positive affirmation is a statement, phrased in terms of the here and now, of what you want to bring about as though it had already happened. Instead of saying, 'I will become,' you say: 'I am.' And, to your surprise at first, you do become whatever it is you are affirming. So affirming: 'I accept and welcome change,' enables you to do so. Affirming: 'I let go of the past and embrace the present,' brings that about. The Australian Bush Essence Bottlebrush will help you to accept and embrace necessary change and make the major transitions of life. Affirmations can be written or spoken. They should be repeated two or three times a day for a week or so, until the change is apparent. You can stick them up over the sink or your desk, or any place where you will see them and be reminded of your intention.

▶ *ToDo*

Look at all the things on your list that you need to accept. Make yourself a positive affirmation for each one. Spend a few moments each day repeating the affirmations.

Reparation

Part of the 'unfinished business' menopause brings to the surface is regret for things done, or not done. If this involves another person, then it is never too late to make reparation. You may like to perform some service, send flowers, write a letter — whatever you feel is appropriate.

If you are no longer in touch with that person, then choose a symbolic means of reparation or dedicate an act of kindness to their memory. You may like to give a donation—money or time—to an appropriate charity, or send flowers to a lonely old lady. Do whatever feels good to you.

▶ *ToDo*

Look at the past action for which you wish to make reparation.

What would be an appropriate act now?

Is it possible to make it directly to the person concerned?

If so, do so. If not, find an agreeable substitute.

Forgiveness

Accepting someone's forgiveness, or giving forgiveness yourself, brings about an inner healing. It cleanses your spirit. If it is possible, and appropriate, try to talk to the person concerned. You may find it easier to write it down first and then read it. If you are seeking forgiveness, set out your reasons. If you are giving forgiveness, explain why you feel this is necessary. The person does not have to be physically present; you can talk to a photograph or a mental picture. (If you are forgiving yourself, then you can act both parts using two chairs, one for the part of you that is forgiving and the other for the part that is receiving the forgiveness. Move between the two as appropriate.) If you are a religious person, then you can pray for forgiveness, or go to confession and receive absolution.

There may be non-specific things for which you feel you yourself need forgiveness. If so, a visualisation can help you.

▶ *ToDo*

Settle yourself comfortably in a chair and close your eyes. Picture in front of yourself a small pink ball of light. This light grows bigger and stronger until you are totally surrounded by it. It is a loving presence, offering you forgiveness. Let the forgiveness soak through to every particle of your being.

When you have accepted all the forgiveness you can absorb, let the light slowly pull back into the small pink ball. Place it in your heart.

Then slowly return your awareness to the room.

Releasing baggage

Everyone carries emotional baggage that they have long since finished with but forgot to let go of. It is possible to release this baggage without having to know exactly what it is.

▶ *ToDo*

Sit with your eyes closed. You are going to be given an invisible hoovering.

Sense a benign presence coming to you with a vacuum cleaner to remove all the emotional baggage you have been carrying unawares. The hoovering starts at the top of your head. Then it slowly moves down the front of your body, paying special attention to your solar plexus and lower belly. When it reaches your feet, the benign presence moves round to your back, moving slowly upwards. It pays special attention to your shoulders, neck and base of the skull. When it reaches the top of your head again, the benign presence switches the vacuum cleaner off. You may feel some 'holes' in your energy field where you have let go of baggage. The benign presence removes any burdens your shoulders are carrying, leaving them free and unfettered.

Then the benign presence passes healing energy from the top of your head right through your body down to your toes. This healing energy cleanses, purifies and revitalises all the parts of your being that were holding on to old emotional baggage.

When this process has finished, notice how much lighter you feel. How much clearer.

Thank the benign presence for its help. Then bring your attention back into the room and open your eyes.

If you find that there are any other feelings or unfinished business connected with menopause on your list, you can adapt any of the above techniques. Affirmations, for instance, are extremely good when making any kind of change and 'finding the benefit' can be helpful in recognising the positive side of any regrets you may have uncovered.

Mood Medicine

Both flower essences and homoeopathy can help to bring about a change in how you feel. You can overcome fear, change how you perceive yourself, dissolve negative feelings such as resentment, find new confidence, etc, with just a few drops of the appropriate flower essence taken twice a day for two to four weeks. You may well find that you feel worse before you feel better. If you persevere and work through the emotions, allowing them to rise up into your awareness, acknowledging each one as how you feel, then they will soon dissipate or change to a more constructive feeling.

▶ *FactFile*

▶ *Flower essences for emotional transformation:*

Buttercup (Cal) counteracts low self-worth and a sense of being undervalued.

Hibiscus (Cal) is the remedy for lack of sexual warmth and vitality.

Henna (Cal) helps philosophical acceptance of life changes and attunement to inner wisdom.

Mallow (Cal) and *Peach-Flowered Tea-Tree* (Bush) overcome fear of ageing, conferring a sense of dignity.

Wild Oat (Bach) is useful in cases where you feel unfulfilled and dissatisfied with life so far and have now reached a crossroads, not knowing which direction to take.

Illawarra Flame Tree (Bush) counteracts feelings of rejection.

Wisteria (Bush) heals sexual abuse.

Crab Apple (Bach) cleanses feelings of self-loathing.

Confidessence (Bush) helps restore confidence.

▶ **Anger**

Holly (Bach) is useful where anger is accompanied by jealousy, bitterness, envy, rage and hatred.

Mountain Devil (Bush) clears anger, hatred, suspicion and the holding of grudges and brings about unconditional love.

▶ **Resentment**

Dagger Hakea (Bush) is helpful in cases where there is resentment and bitterness, particularly towards partners and close family. It opens the door to forgiveness.

Willow (Bach) helps to dissolve resentment and bring about healing.

▶ **Fear**

Dagger Hakea (Bush) helps where there is a fear of lack. It is also an excellent remedy for the emotionally closed personality, opening the heart to love, joy and expression of feelings.

Aspen (Bach) is for anxiety and irrational fears of unknown origin.

Cherry Plum (Bach) is for fear of being unable to control negative thoughts and feelings.

Mimulus (Bach) is for fears of specific origin (including of death or being alone).

Red Chestnut (Bach) is helpful for when the fear is for the well-being of others.

Rock Rose (Bach) is for panic, fear and terror.

▶ **Grief**

Sturt Desert Pea (Bush) gently releases deep hurt and sadness following any kind of loss.

Fringed Violet (Bush) releases deep shock if it has been part of loss.

Sturt Desert Rose (Bush) clears guilt associated with grief.

▶ **Rejection**

Illawarra Flame Tree (Bush) is helpful if you are feeling an overwhelming sense of rejection.

▶ **Low self-esteem**

Five Corners (Bush) is the remedy to take if you are suffering from low self-esteem and a feeling of being crushed by others.

▶ **Homoeopathy**

Ignatia 200c helps to bring old grief to the surface and release it.

References

1   WDDTY, Vol. 7 No. 8

▶ *Jottings*

Sexuality

Sexuality is far more than just sexual activity.[2] It has a powerful feeling dimension. Your sexuality is bound up with how you perceive yourself as a woman, how comfortable you are with your own feelings, and how much of these feelings you can share. If feelings are blocked, then you cannot feel comfortable about loving. Your body will feel somehow starved, strangely numb despite any amount of physical stimulation. Emotional blockage has physical repercussions. If you are afraid and do not trust (yourself or your partner) then you cannot let go enough to reach orgasm. If your heart and emotions are not involved, then sex is somehow empty and without meaning. Lack of intimacy is behind many an apparent loss of libido. If you are someone who finds a sexual identity in how you look, or in being admired, then the physical changes that accompany menopause can bring about a profound depression on the feeling level. This is so whether or not you have an ongoing sexual relationship.

Emotion and sex are inextricably linked, and so too is the past. Your previous experience will inevitably colour your sexuality and your emotional response. Emotions that may arise during any kind of sexual interaction, including intimacy, are joy, anger, guilt, sadness and anxiety. If you have experienced abuse or painful relationships, this will be reflected in your sexuality. (The Australian Bush Essences *Wisteria, Fringed Violet* and *Billy Goat Plum* can help here.)

You may never have known what you really want in a sexual relationship. So often early experiences are furtive, forceful, based on ignorance. There is much confusion around sex and sexuality in young adulthood. Your partner said one thing, your mother another. On the other hand, having become a liberated woman, you may have been so busy chasing an orgasm that you missed out on the pleasure of close personal interaction — intimacy. So exploring your emotions and allowing yourself to feel are essential if you are to express yourself fully through your sexuality — as is listening to your body. Your body knows what it needs. It will tell you by physical responses and much more subtle sensations if you are being nourished by your loving. There may be days when all you want is a hug, maybe even just someone to touch. There may be days when what you need is raw, passionate sex. If you are listening to your needs, then on the days when you want to be touched, if you do not have a partner who is willing to do this for you, you can go for a massage. If what you want is sex, pure and simple, then the remedy is in your own hands. If what you want is a loving, sharing relationship, then learn to say so. Partners cannot be expected to be mind readers. Learning to communicate your emotional needs is vital for good loving.

Loving yourself

If you are unable to love yourself, then you are unable to love someone else or to accept their love for you. Loving yourself has generally been socially unacceptable, especially for women who grew up in the 1950s. Loving yourself was frowned on as somehow self-centred, hedonistic, egotistical and 'not quite nice'. Children, including teenagers, were brought up to be 'seen and not heard'. Parents expected their children to do as they were told, schools frowned on individuality, and society expected girls to grow up and marry. Women were, on the whole, expected to 'save themselves' for The Man. The swinging sixties came along and threw all that to one side, but many women now reaching menopause were impregnated throughout childhood with the ideal of a specific kind of womanhood and found it difficult to shake it off. Even when not-conforming became the norm, there was still the lingering question: 'What will they think of me?' So deep down inside there were doubts: 'Am I a good enough person?' 'Am I worth loving?' Much of the old programming remained — and may still do so.

Menopause can be when all that ends. It is a time to get to know yourself, and to find out you are really a rather nice person after all. A time to pamper yourself, and meet your own needs for a change. A time when being alone does not necessarily mean being lonely, because you have yourself for company.

▶ ToDo

Tick the responses that apply to you:

	true	false
Loving myself is selfish	☐	☐
I should serve other people, put them first	☐	☐
I'm not important	☐	☐
I'm not worth bothering about	☐	☐
I don't deserve to be loved	☐	☐
I don't like myself	☐	☐

If you feel that some or all of these statements are true, then you may not be valuing yourself quite as much as you could do. This may be because of old programming, a situation which can be reversed.

Take each statement which you felt was true and try to turn it around, to see the other side of it — the face that would enable you to love yourself. And then make a positive affirmation of the new view. So, if you said yes to 'Loving myself is selfish', turn this around to 'Loving myself is the greatest gift I can give myself'. Use this as a positive affirmation: 'I am lovable and loved'. If you felt you did not deserve love, then turn it around to 'I deserve love'. Practise these affirmations every day.

Loving yourself means accepting yourself, warts and all. It means being non-judgemental and totally accepting of yourself — being happy with who you are. When you love yourself, you are able to care for yourself, to nurture yourself, to meet your own needs without feeling guilty. You have a strong sense of self: of who you are. If you love yourself in this way, then you accept your weaknesses, your foibles, as part of you, just as your strengths are. They are a part that you might want to improve on, but nevertheless they are OK because they are you.

Feeling good

▶ *ToDo*

Set aside time for yourself each day. In that time, do something that makes you feel good. Begin by writing in your special book at least five good points about yourself. How warm and caring you are, how good you are at . . . , how much better you are at coping these days, how much more you are in touch with your emotions. Whatever makes you feel good. Then think of what you need that would nurture you, make you feel pampered and cared for. This might be a luxurious bath, it might be eating some chocolates that you have bought specially, it might be doing some yoga. Do this with joy and do not feel guilty for taking the time. Affirm to yourself that you deserve it.

The Other Dimension of the Heart: Intimacy

An intimate relationship is a close, warm, personal one where you share your thoughts and feelings freely. Where you are known, and know, the other person deeply. An intimate relationship is based on trust and openness, not on symbiosis or dependency. Such relationships are often sexual, but they do not need to be. Your most intimate relationship may be with a girlfriend or your dog. However, a sexual relationship without intimacy will never be wholly fulfilling. Many people think that because they share their life with someone, using the same bathroom, sleeping together, having sex together, they must be intimate. But this is not necessarily so. Unless a sharing of feelings is also involved, the relationship is not intimate.

Do you have an intimate relationship?

► *ToDo*

Tick the boxes that apply to you:

Do you share everything with your partner? ☐

Can you tell your partner exactly how you are feeling? ☐

Do you know how your partner is feeling? ☐

Can you say no to your partner? ☐

Can you ask for a cuddle if this is what you need? ☐

Can you express your sexual needs? ☐

Can you take time to be on your own? ☐

Your partner instinctively knows what you need ☐

Do you express your anger to your partner? ☐

Misunderstandings rarely arise ☐

If you tick all or most of these boxes, then you have an intimate relationship. If you tick very few, then intimacy can be learned. Look at what you have not ticked. Does fear of expressing anger hold you back? Lack of trust in yourself or your partner shows itself in not allowing your anger to surface. A good argument in which you express all your feelings can be very intimate indeed, providing you *are* expressing your feelings, not simply blaming your partner for them. Are you afraid to express your need for solitude, or for closeness without sex? Maybe you need to learn to say: 'This is what I need.' Where there is real love, your partner will hear you and meet those needs. If there is no real love, then this is a different issue entirely. You may need to look at whether the relationship gives you enough benefit to make it worth continuing. Is it based on financial or emotional dependence, a fear that you cannot manage on your own? Do you stay because you have nowhere else to go? Do you feel the children need you to be together? Has it simply become a habit? These are questions that you may need to talk over with someone — a friend or counsellor. They could well be at the bottom of many of your menopausal disturbances. You could also explore whether you and your partner could make it a more intimate relationship. Is there something there that is worth saving?

Opening your heart

If you do want intimacy, then you need to keep your heart open. No matter what happens, you need to stay in a place of loving acceptance. To hear and accept what is said to you without taking it as a personal attack or affront. To be open in your response and in your own sharing of feelings. There is no room for criticism, judgement, defensiveness or over-sensitivity in intimacy. This does not mean, however, that you have to accept everything that is thrown at you, or allow yourself to be walked all over or abused in any way. Intimacy includes saying no, setting boundaries, expressing anger when it is appropriate. If you are afraid to do this, then your heart is not open.

▶ *ToDo*

Close your eyes. Take your attention to your heart. Be aware of its beat. Be aware of how it permeates your physical body through the pulse. Then be aware of the other dimension of the heart — the subtle, feeling part.

Focus on your heart chakra just above and between your breasts. Picture it as a flower. You may find that when you first see it, it is like a tightly furled bud that needs to open gently. Or you may find that it is a fully opened flower. Its colour will probably be pink. Let your heart open fully. Then see pink light around it, streaming out from it. You can control the flow of energy, either holding it around your heart to keep it open but protected from unwanted intrusion, or letting it flow out to a person with whom you are sharing intimacy. Practise this for a few moments.

Deliberately bring to mind the person with whom you wish to share intimacy. Picture them at their worst, in a bad moment. Then let the pink light stream out to surround them with loving acceptance. Do nothing else, just let the light be there.

When you are ready, let the flow of energy gently break off and encompass your own heart once more.

Slowly return your awareness to the room and open your eyes.

Then, when you are with that person, open your heart once more. Let the light stream out to surround them, forming a bridge between you. Practise saying what you are feeling. Practise listening to what they feel without judging it or feeling you have to respond personally. Ask your partner to open their heart too.

You may like to buy yourself a piece of rose quartz crystal, either polished or as a chunk, and use this to remind yourself to keep that heart open.

▶ *FactFile*

Essences for intimacy

Karma Clear (Findhorn) releases the past and helps in understanding the deep-seated cause of problems.

Spiritual Marriage (Findhorn) brings about harmony, union and the joy of right relationship.

Relationship Essence (Bush) enhances the quality of intimate relationships.

Sexuality Essence (Bush) heals sexual and relationship trauma. Brings about an openness to sexuality and touch. Aids physical and emotional intimacy.

Bush Gardenia (Bush) renews passion and interest in the relationship.

Wedding Bush (Bush) aids commitment.

Billy Goat Plum (Bush) releases shame and enhances body image.

Wisteria (Bush) heals abuse and overcomes frigidity leading to gentleness and openness in relationships.

Pink Mulla Mulla (Bush) heals loners who feel isolated.

Sexual Harmony (DA) brings about a light-hearted balance and harmony in sexual relationships.

As your mental attitude to sexuality can also affect your relationships, you will find more work to do on page 193 onwards.

References

1   Study quoted in *Proof*, Vol.1, 1996
2   *Menopause Matters*, Judy Hall & Robert Jacobs, Element Books, 1994

V: Mind

Change is fear of unknown things approaching

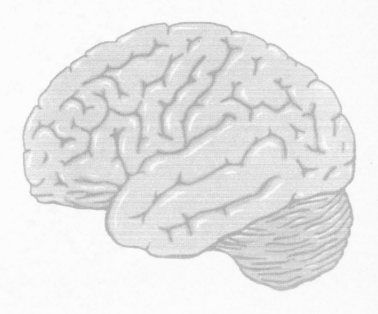

Menopause: All in the Mind?

Despite what science would have us believe, the mind is much more than a by-product of the brain. Mind is intellect, but it is also instinct and intuition. A repository for beliefs and mores, it is influenced by attitudes and feelings. It has many levels. The conscious mind is the tip of an iceberg: below it sits the unconscious mind and the collective unconscious which links to ancestral memories. The mind can condition our experiences. Much of what accompanies menopause comes from the deeper levels of the mind.

As we have seen, back in the 19th century, menopause came to be looked on as a disease. Not only was it a physical event, it was also regarded as a mental disturbance. The Victorian gynaecologist Edward Tilt saw menopause as 'a gradual loss of feminine grace'. In his mind it led to mental diseases, morbid irrationality, hysteria, melancholia and an impulse towards drink, kleptomania and murder.[1] It is not surprising that many women fear that menopause indicates an inevitable decline into senile dementia or worse.

It is this kind of attitude that has created much of the modern disease. Women have been indoctrinated to expect the worst. Menopausal women have been figures of fun, or have been pitied. Unfortunately society tends to reinforce this by accepting the stereotyped picture of a midlife woman as being 'past it'. In a society which values youth and beauty above age and wisdom, encroaching age is seen as something to be feared. Much of the advertising for HRT focuses on the aspect of halting age, holding back the 'inevitable decay'. Unfortunately, some of the new 'natural' hormones are also being marketed as 'the fountain of youth', reinforcing the prejudice against growing older.

Your own attitudes to the menopause, and to ageing, may well affect not only how you view menopause but also how you experience it. If your mother suffered her way through menopause, then at a sub-conscious level you will have assimilated the thought: 'This is how it is.' At the first sign of a hot flush, confusion, dizziness, you will think: 'Here I go; I knew it would happen to me. It's all downhill from here.' So identifying all those underlying thoughts about menopause can help you to reframe how you expect to experience it. This in turn influences your actual experience.

Menopause Myths

Not only does society have its myths about menopause, families do too. Go back to that exercise where you wrote down everything about meno-pause including what you were told by your family or friends (pages 21 & 22). Read it again. Maybe you can recall more of what the matriarchs in your family passed on to you — not all of it will have been spoken of openly, much might have been hinted at. Whether you are aware of it or not, this is your own menopausal myth. It will have its roots in attitudes to menstruation, for so long known as 'the curse'. This, along with pain in childbirth, is supposed to be God's punishment to women for daring to be independent and think for themselves. It was Eve, after all, who told Adam to eat that apple. According to some sources she was offered it by Lilith, primal woman and Adam's first wife. Other sources say that it was Sophia, pre-existing feminine wisdom, who persuaded her to give up her state of ignorance. Eve was put in touch with her instinctual knowing, and ate the fruit of the tree of knowledge. In other words, she balanced instinct and intellect, to become whole.

The Old Testament God made the whole business of womanhood 'unclean'. Much earlier, as we shall see, menstruation was looked on as sacred and magical, a gift from the Goddess. It was only woman who could bleed without being cut, and who lived to tell the tale. Wise blood was honoured — it held the secret of life and creation. And those who retained their wise blood were likewise honoured.

▶ ToDo

How do you view menopause?

It is a time when my function as a woman ends ☐

Sex life ceases or diminishes ☐

My sexual desirability fades ☐

A release from 'the curse' ☐

A time of inevitable mental and physical decline ☐

Something new, exciting and challenging ☐

A time when I can come into my own ☐

A new opportunity ☐

A new freedom to be sexually adventurous ☐

Something that will give more time for me ☐

Clearly the first five present a negative view of menopause while the second five are much more positive and forward-looking.

When you have worked through this book, you might like to take the time to write your own menopausal myth, one that is positive and life-enhancing and which could be passed on to your children (the Australian Bush Essence *Turkey Bush* aids creativity and could help you with this).

Inherited beliefs

If you have inherited some particularly pernicious and life-destroying myths, then you can reframe these into a more positive view. You need to separate your original list into beliefs that work for you and those that do not.

▶ *ToDo*

Go through your list of beliefs about menopause. Write down any others that come to mind. Tick any that you emphatically agree with and put a cross against any that you feel are negative.

You may well find that some of the beliefs you agree with are negative but have a 'pay-off'. Pay-offs are hidden benefits. So, if you have never really enjoyed a sexual relationship, believing that midlife is the time when sexual attractiveness and desire diminish will have the pay-off of less sex (assuming your partner shares your belief, that is). That may actually be what you need. A time free from the pressure to be sexual may allow you to opt for celibacy as a positive choice. But if you forgo that pay-off and learn to enjoy your sexuality, then the belief will change. You can use positive affirmations to help you make the change: 'I am a sexually desirable woman who enjoys a full sexual relationship.' (You can also use your menopause diary to chart when your sexual desire is at its peak and when you need time alone. In which case being able to state that need for solitude, and to sleep alone if necessary, will help you to enjoy sexual contact more when you do feel like it.)

You may find that the thought, 'I'm past it,' has the hidden pay-off that you don't have to make an effort any more. This may point to a deeper truth. You need simply to be yourself, as you are. Indeed, you may need to give yourself permission to take time out, to give yourself a space to be who you are. When you give up struggling, trying to do or be, then you can allow things simply to be as they are. Your affirmation can be: 'I am exactly the way I should be.' You can also affirm that all possibilities are open to you.

Try to identify as many pay-offs as possible in the negative views you have expressed about menopause. Think about these. What is the hidden benefit? What are they telling you about what you need? Can you reframe them into positive affirmations or give yourself what you need?

Learning to say 'No'

You may well discover from the work you have done that your greatest difficulty is that you always do what other people want or expect from you. You cannot say no. Some of the symptoms you have may occur for this reason. It is a way of giving you the opportunity of learning to say no. There are different kinds of no. There is the no that says: 'I don't feel like that at the moment'; the no that says: 'I have some fear around that but I might be persuaded'; and the no that says: 'Absolutely, categorically not.' When you are learning to say no, it helps if you yourself know what kind of no you mean. You can then communicate that clearly. Practising first helps! Very often, saying yes when you mean no comes out of family or societal pressure to conform, to 'do your duty', to 'be a good person'. If you find there is something of this in your no-saying, then it can help to go over the 'Loving yourself' exercise on page 169, as saying no is much easier when you are not looking to someone else for approval all the time.

▶ *ToDo*

Think about something you are doing that you would rather not be doing. Something to which you felt it impossible to say no:

1. Is it a longstanding pattern? Are you giving in
   to family pressure, for instance? ☐

2. Is it something that you don't feel like doing right now,
   but could maybe feel more like doing later? ☐

3. Are you hesitant about it because you are afraid
   you are not capable, or you won't enjoy it? ☐

4. Is it something that you really do not want to do? ☐

5. Are you afraid of what people will think if you say no? ☐

Having decided which kind of no you want to say, think about how you can go about this. It may be enough simply to say no and mean it. But you may need to communicate the reason behind your no. The 'three-part assertion message' helps you communicate without attaching blame. The first part sets out the when or what of the situation, the second what happens, and the third how you feel about it. You can also add a fourth part: what you would like to do or what you would like to change. So, taking the example about sex, you could say: 'When I have sex when I don't feel like it, I get sore, and that makes me feel abused. I would like to have sex at a time in my cycle when I feel ready for it and can enjoy it too.'

If you have identified a need to have your own space, you might also want to say: 'When I'm suffering from night sweats it makes things worse to be sharing a bed, as it is hotter with someone else there. I need to throw the bedclothes off, and often I need to change my nightwear and the sheets. I worry about disturbing your sleep and so I get anxious, which makes the sweats worse. I feel I need to have my own bed (or bedroom) so that I can take care of my needs. This doesn't mean we can't have cuddles or sex any more. I would still like to come into your bed and share time with you.'

Write down exactly how you are going to communicate your no. Next, picture yourself saying this and the person you are speaking to hearing it and accepting it in a loving way. Then say it to them in person.

You can also practise looking in the mirror and saying no until you look as though you mean it and convince yourself you can do it.

If necessary, refer back to physicalising anger (page 153) and practise stamping and shouting, 'No,' to dissipate any anger before you communicate with the person concerned.

Irrational fears

An irrational fear is a fear without a logical cause. Irrational fears have their source in the mind. They often stem from the past and are lodged in the 'old brain' at the back of the head. Sometimes these irrational fears are totally in the mind — for instance, the fear that someone will leave or die. At other times they have a paralysing effect on the whole body, and may have a particular trigger such as an animal. This is a phobia. You will find under Fear (pages 154–6) appropriate remedies to help you release yourself from these feelings but *Grey Spider Orchid* (Bush) is appropriate where the fear has reached phobic proportions (take several times a day for a month). Looking at your fear can help you to handle it and may also show you where it is coming from — although the essence of an irrational fear is that it may not have an accessible source. If your fear-state and paralysis are overwhelming, then help from a psychologist or hypnotherapist would help you overcome it.

▶ *ToDo*

Write down as fully as possible exactly what it is you fear (do this for each fear). Does it concern another person?

How long have you had this fear?

What kind of situations bring the fear up?

Is there a specific trigger?

Have you shared this fear with anyone?

Your fear may well have started from a sensible base, a genuine worry, and was something that protected you. But if it is now irrational it will have got out of hand. Whilst you can spend time exploring the fear and eventually finding out where it came from, it can be most helpful to learn to 'switch off' the fear. If you know what the trigger is, then the following exercise can be carried out whenever the trigger is present. If you are not sure what triggers it, practise the exercise from time to time throughout the day. The more you do it, the stronger it will become in its effect of 'switching off' the fear. It can be helpful to take a dose of Grey Spider Orchid before doing this exercise:

Sit with your eyes closed. Breathe gently and let yourself relax for a few minutes.

Go back to the last time you had the fear. Let yourself feel how it was, how your body responded, how your breathing and heart rate changed.

Then slowly take five deep, even and calm breaths. Notice the effect it has on your fear. Take two more breaths.

Choose some unobtrusive gesture that you can make to switch off your fear such as putting your thumb and forefinger together. Tell yourself that this will switch off the fear when you say to yourself: 'Calm and relaxed.' Keep breathing calmly and evenly. Practise the gesture a few times.

Then, keeping your breathing going, think of your fear again. This time, as soon as you think of it, make the gesture and say: 'Calm and relaxed.' You will feel the fear switch off.

Practise this a few times. Then simply practise the gesture and the affirmation.

Open your eyes and practise it a few more times.

Remember to practise several times a day. Then, when you need it, make the gesture and breathe slowly and calmly, saying to yourself: 'Calm and relaxed.' The fear will subside. Eventually the fear will not even be there.

Fear of ageing

Sometimes the irrational fear may be of death and ageing. We live in a society that does not value older women and many people fear the unknown. But it may be a more rational fear. Perhaps you have a history of heart disease in the family. You may have seen older members of the family slowly crumble from osteoporosis, or become housebound with arthritis, or face increasing senility. As a result of your fear, you may be steadfastly refusing to face the onset of midlife change. Worry and anxiety cause stress, which adds to the probability of physical and mental decline, and certainly does nothing to halt it. It helps to recognise that none of these things are an inevitable consequence of menopause. There are a great many women who live to ripe old age and thoroughly enjoy it. If you pay attention to your diet and exercise properly, if you live a fulfilled life, if you use natural remedies to prevent the ravages of age from taking hold, then there is no need to fear old age. Putting some practical measures in place, including making financial provision if this is part of your worries, is the best prevention there is. If you find yourself worrying obsessively about old age, take *Mallow* (Cal) or *Peach-Flowered Tea-Tree* (Bush) to help you move towards that period of your life with dignity rather than fear.

Change how you view things

Menopause can be a time of enormous possibility, of releasing unlimited potential. It is the point in your life when your hopes and dreams can become reality.

▶ *ToDo*

List as many things as possible that you would like to do.

Then look at what is holding you back. Is it your belief in yourself, fear, circumstances? A little ingenuity may be called for, but you can make it work. With each one, make a positive decision to get started. To believe in yourself enough to do it. Set a date, and stick to it.

When you are in control of your own life, then you find that your view of the menopause naturally changes. It becomes an exciting place, challenging but fun. A time of change, yes, of transition, of movement into something different. 'An unpredicted life now shaped.'

Midlife crisis

If you have discovered that you are having a midlife crisis, now is the time to do something constructive. If your crisis is related to specific events, having come this far through the book will have given you tools to handle the situation and to make changes. If your crisis is one of meaning and identity, then the Spirit section of the book will help you explore further, as will getting in touch with your intuitive self (a few pages further on). Make a note now of anything you need to come back to and look at later.

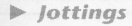 **Jottings**

Mind medicine

Ginkgo Biloba

Ginkgo is known throughout the world as the 'memory tree'. It stimulates the circulation in the brain and enhances memory and brain function. It is one of the finest aids there is to clarity of thought and improved memory. The concentrated extract taken in water works fastest. It can also be taken in tablet form or as a tincture. Ginkgo should not be taken for prolonged periods of time. Take for six months at the most and then have a break of one to three months.

Agnus Castus

In the 3x homoeopathic potency, Agnus Castus can improve memory and word blindness (making mistakes in speech, missing words out, putting the wrong one in or completely forgetting what you were about to say). It also relieves anxiety and confusion.

Kali Carb

In homoeopathic potency, Kali Carb is extremely effective for poor memory and for word blindness. It can be obtained from homoeopathic chemists or suppliers and is effective in the 6x or 30x potency.

▶ *Flower essences*

Isopogon (Bush) is an aid against poor memory and for the retrieval of forgotten skills.

Boronia (Bush) brings clarity of thought and mental calmness; clears obsessive thoughts.

Bauhinia (Bush) overcomes resistance to necessary change.

Bush Fuchsia (Bush) synchronises the left and right brain.

Henna (Cal) helps the philosophical acceptance of change and in accessing wisdom.

Mallow (Cal) and *Peach-Flowered Tea-Tree* (Bush) overcome fear of ageing and confer a sense of dignity.

Turkey Bush (Bush) opens the mind to creative possibilities, corrects left-brain dominance and enhances creativity.

Sundew and *Red Lily* (Bush) compensate for right-brain dominance.

Sunshine Wattle (Bush) overcomes expectations based on negative experiences in the past.

Cognisessence (Bush) gives enhanced mental clarity.

Boronia and *Bush Iris* (Bush) help in creative visualisation.

Grey Spider Orchid (Bush) overcomes phobias.

Creative Visualisation

Some of the exercises in this book use creative visualisation. This is a simple process of using your imagination to bring about change. It uses 'mind pictures', what you see with your inner eye. However, you may not actually see anything when doing a visualisation. Some people are non-visual. If this happens for you, then 'act as if' — try to feel what is going on rather than forcing something to happen. Visualisation improves with practice. The more relaxed you are, the less you strive to form the images, the easier it is. Music can help with relaxation and visualisation and there are many suitable tapes available. You may also find that looking up to the point above and between the eyebrows, with your eyes closed, helps the images to form. Believing in what you are doing is the most essential part of visualisation. It triggers the power of your mind to bring things into being. Visualisation is a right-brain activity.

▶ *FactFile*

▶ *Enhancing visualisation*

Be as relaxed as possible.

Do not try to force images.

Look up to the point above and between your eyebrows.

'Act as if' something is happening.

Practise.

Believe in it.

Boronia and *Bush Iris* (Bush) help images to form.

White Chestnut (Bach) and *Isopogon* (Bush) stop 'mind chatter'.

In Two Minds?

The brain can be seen as having four sections: the two hemispheres and the front and rear brain. The rear part holds old memories, both personal and inherited. It is this part we work with when we consider our attitude to menopause, especially the ingrained beliefs we hold. When we look at how we think, we work with the right and left hemispheres. The phrase 'in two minds' is very apt. Each side thinks and perceives in a different way and these can be complementary to each other or light years apart. The way in which each side of the brain perceives reality is unique.

The left brain is logical and rational, the right brain emotional and intuitive. Where the left brain reasons things through carefully and then forms a theory, the right brain takes a great intuitive leap — and can rarely explain how it got there. Most people use one side of their brain more than the other. Artists and other creative people use their right brain. Scientists and administrators use their left brain. Women tend towards right-brain dominance. Men are usually left-brain dominant. In a few people the two sides of the brain balance each other and interact.

Menopausal women often experience difficulty with words: losing them, muddling them up, substituting others. But your hands know exactly what you mean; their gestures indicate what your tongue cannot say. This is because your tongue tends to be linked to the left brain and your hands to the right brain. As a result of fluctuating hormone levels, one side of the brain is being stimulated more than the other. This is part of the natural development of brain synthesis — a process menopausal women are intended to undergo. It is the linking of the two halves that produces the post-menopausal wise woman.

► **ToDo**

Is your thinking:

Linear	☐	Holistic	☐
Word-orientated	☐	Non-verbal	☐
Logical	☐	Intuitive	☐
Analytical	☐	Towards synthesis	☐
Intellectual	☐	Imaginative	☐
Reasoned	☐	Idealistic	☐
Symbolic	☐	Metaphoric	☐
Judgemental	☐	Feeling-orientated	☐
Time-orientated	☐	Outside time	☐
Sequential	☐	Boundless	☐
Abstract	☐	Spatially perceptive	☐
Categorical	☐	Insightful	☐
Theoretical	☐	Experiential	☐
Goal-orientated	☐	Process-orientated	☐
'Masculine'	☐	'Feminine'	☐
Do your hands stay still when you talk?	☐	Do you talk with your hands?	☐

If you tick more boxes in the left-hand column, then your thinking is mainly left-brain. If you tick more boxes on the right, it is more right-brain. (But note that if you are left-handed the hemispheres may be opposite — that is, the left-hand side thinks in a right-brain way.) An equal number of ticks on both sides indicates a left-right synthesis. You can confirm this by a simple exercise:

Close your eyes and relax. Let yourself become attuned to your mental energies. Draw your attention away from the outside world and into your self. Take your attention up to your head. Does one side feel bigger than the other. Is there a lot of activity going on in one side? Does one side feel smaller, somehow emptier? Does the energy radiate out from one side only?

Now make a mental shopping list of things to buy when you are next at the store. Notice which side of your head feels active.

Then think of a point which is moving ever inwards to create a spiral. Try to visualise it in your mind's eye. The point moves from the outside of a circle, going round and round in ever-decreasing circles until it reaches the centre. Which side of your head feels stimulated now?

You will probably notice that one side of your head does feel much more 'there' than the other. This is the side of the brain that is dominant. When you make your shopping list, you will probably find that the left side seems busier. Creating a spiral uses the right-hand side of the brain.

You can balance the two sides by doing something that uses the less active side. If you are right-brain dominant, then making lists, doing your accounts, reading a map or writing a business letter will stimulate the left brain. If you are left-brain dominant, then painting, listening to music, daydreaming or writing a story will strengthen your right brain. It can also be helpful to deliberately choose a right- or left-brain way of communicating. You can draw, using colours and patterns, for instance, to express feelings when the words of the left brain are inadequate. Or, if you are feeling particularly woolly, you can sit down and make lists to activate the left brain. Eventually, you can instinctively choose either pattern of thought — or both.

You can also bring about a balance or synthesis between the two sides using flower essences (see Mind Medicine) and by a simple visualisation:

▶ ### Uniting your mind

Take your attention to the middle of your head, from your forehead to the back. Immediately below this line is where the two sides of the brain join. Imagine that there is a zigzag line of light from the front of your head to the back. This light joins the two sides of your brain and stimulates the neural pathways that cross between the two. Picture the light flashing along the pathway, uniting the two halves.

You can also work with the goddess Sophia to attune to your intuitive wisdom and use rational thought (see Spirit, pages 211–4).

When the two sides of the brain unite, you have become the wise woman.

The Intuitive Self

Intuition is a function of the mind. It is complementary to intellect but works in the opposite way. It arises from the instinctual side of your being. Instinct is rooted in the collective consciousness, its branches are in nature and its flowering is intuition. Bypassing the logical and rational part of the mind, intuition takes small pieces of knowledge, tiny clues, and makes a great leap forward into new knowing. Intuition is timeless, it can go backwards or project forwards into the future. In ancient times all post-menopausal women were to some extent believed to have the power of inner sight, the ability to peer through the veil that separates the worlds, and so to contact both those who had gone before and what was to come. Women in whom this ability was well developed became the seers and healers for the tribe, the wise women.

The wise woman is a figure of inspiration and intuition. She acts as a mediator between the two worlds: the visible and the invisible, the conscious and the unconscious, the known and the unknown. She is a midwife to the psyche and gives assistance in times of difficult passage, leading women into their own inner 'knowing'. Many of the 'symptoms' experienced as part of the menopause are actually an opening up of intuitive and psychic perception. Headaches (particularly frontal mi-graine) or flashes of light, 'tingling' and crawling of the skin, 'giddiness', precognitive flashes or a sense of 'going out of time' all occur when intuitive development is taking place and may have a hormonal basis.

The witch hunts in historical times actively discouraged women from using these powers but nature keeps on trying to re-establish the developmental pattern. If you can look on this ability as a gift rather than something evil and cursed, then it can enhance your life. You can have your visions and take them out into the world to make them manifest. It is possible to take workshops or classes to open up this intuitive and far-seeing faculty and this will speedily remove the disconcerting 'symptoms'.

Sexuality and the Mind

Psychosexual problems

The origin of psychosexual difficulties lies in the mind, not in the physical body. Psychosexual problems can include loss of libido, vaginal dryness and anorgasmia (the apparent inability to have an orgasm). Such problems arise from ingrained attitudes and beliefs about midlife sexuality. They may create situations which appear to get you what you want, but which, on deeper reflection, are not a positive choice. It is one thing to have decided, for instance, that you do not want to continue sexual activity because this is what is right for you. It is another to have found a way to avoid sex for reasons which are not conscious. Psychosexual difficulties respond to expert counselling but it is possible to look at some of the underlying causes yourself.

▶ *FactFile*

Studies have shown that loss of libido is actually more likely to occur prior to menopause and is more likely to be related to relationship difficulties.[1]

One study showed that loss of libido in menopausal women can be caused by psychological and social factors. The women who experienced difficulties were more likely to be married and their husbands were likely to suffer from erectile impotence. When questioned, the woman said that while an active sex life was important to their husband, it was much less so to them. Many of them felt guilt about their loss of libido and had sex for their husband's sake. This in turn led to resentment. The women were also more likely to be anorgasmic. Another study showed that if a woman with psychosexual loss of libido changed partners, then she would probably experience a return of her libido. It has also been suggested that women who experience most difficulty with menopausal symptoms are those who are not comfortable with their own feminine nature, or who see their identity as so deeply rooted in their reproductive function that they cannot see a life beyond.[2]

Attitudes to sex

If you enjoy sex and have a full and satisfying relationship with your partner, then you are unlikely to experience psychosexual problems during menopause. But if there are underlying, unconscious factors affecting how you view sexual activity then you may well experience difficulties.

▶ *ToDo*

Tick the boxes that apply to you:

Do you believe that enjoying sex is 'not nice'? ☐

Do you think it bad to have sexual needs of your own? ☐

Do you feel complete only when with a partner? ☐

Do you think that sex is only for making babies? ☐

Do you believe that sexual attraction is always based
    on physical appearance? ☐

Do you believe that sexuality is tied to your
    reproductive capacity? ☐

Is your sexual role a passive one? ☐

Do you initiate sex? ☐

Is your sex life based on someone else's needs? ☐

Do fantasy and sensuality have a place in your sex life? ☐

Is there room for lust in your life? ☐

Do you believe sex is only for the young? ☐

Do you believe that masturbation is wrong? ☐

Do you believe sex goes on into old age? ☐

Are you satisfied with your sex life? ☐

Do you have a good relationship with your partner? ☐

Would you like to explore different facets of your sexuality? ☐

By looking at the ticks you can quickly become aware of your basic attitude to sex, identifying whether it is viewed positively or as something 'not nice'. This is so whether you have a fulfilling relationship or not.

If you feel that fantasy, sensuality and lust have no place in your life, then passion will be missing. Your sexual contact will become a habit rather than a pleasure. Boredom is one of the greatest turn-offs. Similarly, if you never initiate lovemaking, then you are probably not attuned to your own inner cycle and may not be ready for sex.

If you believe that sex is only for the young, that it is for procreation, that you are 'past it' by the time you get to fifty, then you are unlikely to give yourself fully to the pleasures of sex and sensuality. You may decide that celibacy is the option for you.

If your relationship with your partner is poor, then you are unlikely to be turned on by sex (see Intimacy, page 170). You may need to see whether the relationship is worth saving or whether it would be better to go your separate ways, or to renegotiate the way in which you live together.

Where there is an attitude of 'sex is only for procreation', then there is likely to be guilt if sexual needs continue beyond fertility. When there is a belief that women should not enjoy sex (a hangover from Victorian days), then sexual desire may be repressed. Equally, if you are with a partner who no longer desires you, then you may feel that it is not right still to have sexual needs. You may have been brought up to believe that sex was your duty, rather than a pleasure.

You may never have realised that sexuality is different from sex (see pages 106–108 and 167–170). You may feel incomplete without a partner. You may be in a heterosexual relationship when your real orientation is towards your own sex, but somehow you feel this is wrong and have not allowed yourself to explore your real needs. On the other hand, in some sub-cultures such as feminism, it has become almost *de rigueur* to have a female partner as a statement of female unity. This may not be satisfying all your emotional needs either. All of these attitudes, and many more, can lead to psychosexual difficulties.

▶ *ToDo*

You may like to go through your list and see if you can reframe negative beliefs and attitudes into positive benefits. For instance, if you have always felt that sex is for procreation, you may find that no longer having to worry about contraception is a turn-on.

Pleasing yourself

If you do not have a partner with whom to enjoy sexual activity, then masturbation will help to keep your vagina healthy. However, here again unconscious attitudes may be blocking your pleasure.

▶ *ToDo*

In your special book, write down all you have been told about masturbation by friends and family. Cover your own previous experience. Was it pleasurable? Or did ignorance or guilt prevent you from enjoying it? Then decide if any of your unconsciously absorbed attitudes, or your own thoughts, will prevent you from enjoying personal pleasure. If so, find a way to reframe these and affirm that it is okay to please yourself.

The inner prude

Have you ever noticed how, when you are just about to really enjoy yourself sexually, an inner voice starts up. It criticises, comments, judges, admonishes. This is the inner prude. It is a compilation of what your parents told you (indeed, many people find that the inner prude appears in the guise of their mother or father), what you have internalised from your own experience, and the attitudes you have been taught by other people such as teachers and well-meaning friends. You may find that your inner prude frowns on noise. Or nakedness. Or fantasy. Or just about anything that makes sex fun. Next time you hear that voice, take note. If you have an understanding partner, it may be possible to do the exercise below at that moment. If not, when you are on your own, try the following visualisation (or just listen to the voice).

► *ToDo*

Sit quietly and close your eyes. Take your mind back to the time when you heard that voice. Picture it in your mind. Where you were, who you were with, what you were doing, what you were wearing — if anything. Re-create it as vividly as possible.

When you begin to hear the voice, picture the figure who goes with it. Look at the figure carefully. Does it remind you of anyone? Then ask the figure to tell you all the messages the prude carries. You may like to ask where they come from.

When you have heard all the messages, explain to your prude how those messages are preventing you from fully expressing yourself through your sexuality, how they get in the way of you taking pleasure in your body. Explain that you are trying to change yourself at a very deep level. Ask the prude to help you in that endeavour.

Then picture yourself making love joyfully (or masturbating) while the prude looks on approvingly. Ask the prude to give you some messages that affirm your new sexual persona. Finally, tell the prude you would like to rename it to affirm your new sexual persona. What name would the figure like?

Then thank the figure for coming to you and slowly return your attention to the room. When you are ready, open your eyes and write down the experience as fully as possible. Did you recognise your prude? What was the new name it gave? Make sure you list the old messages and then alongside them put the new messages. If appropriate, turn the new messages into positive affirmations.

Prude medicine

The Australian Bush Flower Essence **Billy Goat Plum** can help to overcome the inner prude.

References

1   Quoted in *Menopause Matters,* Judy Hall & Dr Robert Jacobs. Element Books, Shaftesbury, 1994.

2. Ibid

VI: Spirit

Change is boundaries dissolved,
space unlimited, reaching stars

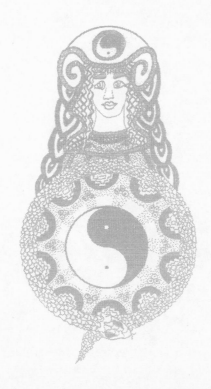

Spirit Power

As well as the physical, emotional and intellectual aspects of your being, you have a spirit. Your spirit is vibrant, inspirational, creative, energetic. It is life-giving. When it leaves, you wither and die. Your spirit is hallowed ground. It is a spark of divine consciousness: the God, or Goddess, within. Without knowledge of your spirit, life becomes joyless and meaningless. Spirit is nourished by connectedness, meditation, communion, joy. Spirit is sacred.

When you recognise your spirit, when you attune to its eternal nature, a marvellous thing happens: you lose your fear of growing old. Death becomes yet another change, one of many transitions you make. It is the fear of death and ageing that drives so much of the menopause machine. HRT is sold on the basis that it will make you feel younger, hold back the years, prevent 'the ravages of time'. In a society that honours how people look, not who they are inside, cronedom is feared. It is the antithesis of youth, so it is not welcomed for its wisdom. Whilst it makes sense to care for your body because it is the vehicle through which your spirit expresses itself, it makes even more sense to nourish your inner being. Your spirit is ageless, eternal. This is where your real power lies.

The sacred quality of women's life has largely been lost in the modern world. Sacredness honours the spiritual in daily life, the numinous presence of a divine power inherent in everything. Personal expression of spirituality is not something separate from everyday life, it is life itself.

Spirituality includes humour, laughter, love and play because these are a vital part of the human experience. Feminine spirituality starts from *knowing*. Knowing is an inner quality, an intuitive wisdom, a connection to all things. You may have forgotten that spirituality is 'a personal odyssey', that you are a spiritual being on a human journey. This results in an increasingly desperate search for meaning and purpose. But that search tends to focus outwards rather than into yourself.

In many ancient traditions women who had passed their childbearing years were offered an opportunity to explore their spirituality. To reconnect to their spirit. They could withdraw from the world, go into retreat, undertake a journey, make a pilgrimage—whatever they needed to find themselves and adjust to their changed role in society. Today, in 'primitive' societies, a change in status follows the lifting of the taboos that surround menstruation. Women are expected to assume responsibility for, and authority over, younger women, instructing them in traditional arts and crafts. They become midwives, matchmakers, traders. They administer the kin system and regulate the social life of the extended family group. They have an important place in the spiritual life of the community. They are the healers, givers of initiation, holy women, 'guardians of the sacred hearth', formal mourners at funeral rites, and they take a full part in ritual ceremonies. All this gives post-menopausal women considerable power in the community.

As a menopausal woman you need this same opportunity to access spirituality and to find a new, post-menopausal role in society. Lack of meaning and purpose can strike most deeply in midlife but this experience can be an essential prerequisite for spiritual growth. It is in the depths of darkness and despair that you find new resources. It is in dissatisfaction with life that you can access a new energy. It is the pain in your life that tells you it is time to find a new way of being.

▶ *FactFile*

▶ ### *Wise blood*

Ancient people believed that women who had passed their menopause were wise women because they retained their menstrual blood. In their world, menstrual blood was magical, potent. It had arcane properties. It was the very stuff of life itself — a gift from the Goddess, a carrier of the spirit. The moon had a strong connection with women's blood. The moon calendar is one of the oldest kinds of calendar in the world. It kept track of women's fertility cycles. The goddesses associated with the moon are related to womb knowledge, an ancient knowing that is older than time.

In many of the ancient wisdom sources it is moon-blood that is both the life-essence of creation and the pathway to spiritual illumination. The Celtic gods obtained their divine nature from the 'red mead' of the faery queen; and the Greeks and many other ancient peoples used 'Hera's red wine' in their sacred mystery rites. If you retained your wise blood, if you passed through the initiation of menopause, then you accessed the hidden knowledge so intimately bound up with woman's menstrual cycle. Those who had moved beyond shedding the sacred blood became the priestesses, seers, healers and midwives leading the tribe to spiritual illumination. They were Wise Women.

This belief may well have a basis in fact. Blood carries the chemical messengers of the body, including hormones. The hormonal changes of menopause can trigger intuition, precognitive dreaming, psychic abilities and spiritual experiences. When the ovaries switch off, the pituitary gland is stimulated to produce large amounts of FSH and LH hormones. The pituitary gland is situated at the 'third eye', a spiritual linkage-point on the forehead. In the East, the third eye is known as the ajna chakra. It is linked to both psychic and spiritual perception. So it appears that women may be intended to become more spiritually aware at menopause, as this is when the third eye becomes activated. Indeed, the message carried by the wise blood may well be: 'Wake up, become illumined.'

Spirit medicine

The gentle touch of flower essences can greatly aid a midlife spiritual transition. They help to align you to your higher purpose, to make contact with your indwelling spirit and with the spiritual energies of the universe. Single flowers or purpose-made essences are available:

Tiger Lily (Cal) aids midlife transition as it makes for inner peace.

Five Corners (Bush) is indicated when there is fear of the awakening psychic powers and intuitive faculties. It is also a remedy for celebrating one's physical being and spiritual essence. It aids self-confidence and recognition of one's inner and outer beauty.

Red Lily (Bush) opens you up to spiritual energies and helps to earth them.

Mint Bush (Bush) prepares you for initiation. It is a good essence to take before guided meditations to meet spiritual parts of yourself.

Spirit Ground (Petaltone) applied to the solar plexus chakra (midriff) helps with many aspects of menopausal transition.

Soul Star (Petaltone) applied to the base chakra (bottom of spine) helps in connecting with and grounding the higher, spiritual self.

White Light (Petaltone) applied to the heart chakra (bottom of breast bone) is an essence of purification and spirituality.

Crack Willow (Green Man), a tree essence, helps you to let go, to allow things to happen. It brings a sense of oneness with the world and communication with the higher self.

Lime (Green Man) helps you to shift levels of consciousness without disorientation.

Plum (Green Man) helps the highest spiritual energies to enter into the material world. It enhances effective use of personal power.

Whitebeam (Green Man) opens you up to the finer levels of creation.

Clear Light (Findhorn) is a combination of Broom, River Findhorn, Wild Pansy, Birch, Scots Pine and Rose Alba. It brings about a peaceful state of mind, mental clarity and brightness. It calms and aligns the heart, body and mind to allow the intuition, higher self and higher mind to be contacted.

Meditation Essence (Bush) was created to deepen spirituality and aid meditation. It contains Fringed Violet, Bush Fuchsia, Bush Iris, Angelsword and Red Lily.

Menopause Essence (SA) enables one to move confidently and calmly into the next chapter of one's life.

Transition (DA) brings peace and ease in times of transition.

Woman of Wisdom (DA) creates balance during menopause and helps support the alchemical process of changing experience into wisdom.

Meditation

Meditation puts you in touch with your spirit.

Meditation is communing with yourself and with the universal spiritual energies (by whatever name you like to call them). Meditation takes you into your inner centre, a place of still, quiet calm. It brings about a change in consciousness, moves you to a 'different space'. There are many different forms of meditation. All require that you enter a relaxed state of mind, but some are active like yoga and tai chi chuan, whilst others are passive like mantra meditations — in which you chant a mantra to yourself, silently or aloud, to switch off the mind and access the spiritual energies. Some meditations use the breath, concentrating on the sensation of the in and out breaths to the exclusion of all else. If you have difficulty concentrating and easily lose focus, you can do guided meditations (like the ones in this book). Drumming and other rhythmic forms of music can change your level of consciousness, as can dance or chanting.

You do not necessarily have to meditate in order to enter a meditative frame of mind. Meditation, like menopause, involves chemical factors. Endorphins, the natural mind tranquillisers, are produced in meditation but they also accompany activities such as running and other forms of exercise. They can be stimulated by rhythmic breathing patterns. 'Active meditations' like tai chi chuan combine several endorphin-raising factors.

One way of increasing your spirituality is to set time aside each day for communion with your inner self. The type of meditation that is best for you depends very much on the type of person you are.

Twenty minutes of meditation a day is the equivalent of two hours' sleep.

Meditation medicine

The Bach Flower Essence *White Chestnut* or the Bush Essence *Boronia* helps to rid the mind of unwanted thoughts during meditation.

▶ *ToDo*

Tick the boxes that apply to you:

Are you active, always rushing around? ☐

Does your mind race at great speed? ☐

Do you find it difficult to concentrate? ☐

Does your mind wander? ☐

Do you find it difficult to quieten your mind? ☐

Are you naturally reflective? ☐

Do you tend to fall asleep if you relax? ☐

Do you find exercise makes you 'high'? ☐

Do you find it easy to visualise? ☐

Do you find movement soothing? ☐

Do you like to chant? ☐

If you find it difficult to switch off, then you may well find one of the mantra meditations helps you to focus your attention in a different way. If you find that your mind wanders rather easily, then maybe an active or guided meditation will suit you better. Or you could use drumming or chanting. If you like movement, then a dance or tai chi meditation could be the thing for you. There are many tapes available, both of guided visualisations and appropriate chants or music, and these can be useful in the initial stages. The relaxation exercise on page 130 is a useful preparation for meditation. When you have become used to entering an altered state of consciousness, you can easily adapt to other methods until you find exactly the right one for you.

The Movers and Shapers of Feminine Experience

Myth helps in accessing feminine spirituality and can show you a new way to be. Myth is inner truth. It presents images and symbols that resonate with your psyche. It is something that belongs to the feminine realm of intuition and knowing. Mythic themes are eternal. Using myth enables your imagination to present you with your own particular truth. Working with the goddesses uses myth to illumine your everyday experience and to access their powerful energies. One of the major reasons for working with the goddesses is to reunite parts of yourself and to reassimilate the ancient wisdom they represent.

Myth reflects archetypal human experience. An archetype is a universal symbol. It is often acted upon unconsciously. The eternally youthful puella (young girl) is, for instance, one archetypal response to ageing. The puella simply refuses to grow up and acts in an insouciant, irresponsible way. She is eternally 'Daddy's little girl'. The old crone is another archetype, and one that often strikes fear into the heart because she has tremendous power and cannot be confined.

The goddesses, and their mythological context, have much to say about feminine psychology. The different facets of woman are portrayed by the different goddesses. The goddesses take you into the depths of the psyche, to a place where integration and healing is possible. The goddesses passed through the basic archetypal experiences of woman, such as birth and loss, rejection and renunciation, abuse and humiliation, passion and jealousy, creation and illumination. They are familiar with the territory, and so act as a guide to any woman undergoing these same passages.

Each goddess represents certain inner drives or qualities, which may be consciously or unconsciously expressed in life. As such, the goddesses can be extremely useful in developing neglected or unrecognised potential, or certain personality traits — such as assertion, confidence, and so on — which would be useful to you. They can act as mentors and inspirers, creating new confidence or instilling a sense of adventure. They have a particular kind of being: lunar consciousness, connection to the cycles of life; instinctual, earthy sexuality; prophetic inner knowledge; and the primal creativity of the Great Mother Goddess. All of this must be reclaimed if you are to make yourself whole.

The influences of the goddesses interweave and alternate throughout life. Midlife especially is a time when repressed or unlived-out facets suddenly emerge, causing 'out of character' behaviour as a new archetype struggles to be born. This usually horrifies friends and family, who put it all down to 'her age, you know'. Menopause is the time when the previously home-loving and passive wife (Demeter, Hestia or Hera) may suddenly start going to classes or workshops to develop a neglected intellect (Athena) or psychic powers (Persephone or the other face of Hestia). Hecate may emerge, urging you into therapy to collect together the scattered parts of yourself. Artemis rising will enable you to holiday alone, or to get a divorce. She was a lesbian goddess and may put you in touch with previously unexplored facets of your sexuality. Aphrodite may come to the fore, resulting perhaps in an affair or a surge of artistic energy. Or in a career woman Demeter may emerge, causing you to fall into the deep depression of the 'empty nest' syndrome.

However, these are opportunities to explore new ways of interacting with the world. Midlife offers the chance to meet the unrecognised parts of yourself and round out your experience. You can consciously choose to attune to a goddess. Say you want to explore your sexuality. Well, Aphrodite, the goddess of love, would be a good start. She is not exactly all sweetness and light; she has her other side too, as you will find out; but she would be a good choice to introduce you to the pleasures of love. But suppose you want to be more adventurous, more independent, more mature. Raunchy even? Then how about Lilith? Adam's first wife could introduce you to a very different side of yourself. Maybe you know someone like her already, someone who could be your role model? If you are trying to develop your own inner wisdom, then Sophia is the mother of all the wisdom goddesses. Attuning to her can put you in touch with your wise self.

Other people often act as useful mirrors for the goddesses. They show the 'missing' part of yourself. Mothers, mothers-in-law and grandmothers, aunts, friends and sisters are all fruitful sources of the goddesses, as are 'superiors' on the career ladder or women who have achieved something you are striving for — they can all be useful role models or mentors as you struggle to express the new energy. Rather than selecting 'acceptable' parts of yourself to present, thereby fragmenting and cutting yourself off from your fundamental nature, you can recognise that 'all this is me'. You then return to a state of integration and wholeness which encompasses the totality of your female nature.

Each culture has its own goddesses. You will have goddess myths with which you will particularly resonate, even though this may be at the level below consciousness. You may find yourself drawn to a particular tradition: American Indian, Celtic, Egyptian, Greek, Scandinavian, etc. Many women find that images of the Goddess emerge spontaneously in their dreams during this time of transition and they can work with them. Your dream diary will help you to keep track of your own special links.

▶ *FactFile*

▶ *Images of the Goddess*

Maidens, old crones, mirrors, cauldrons, spindles, looms, bows, sickles, double-headed axes, moons, grain, pomegranates, caverns, wells, bees, serpents, spiders, cows, eggs, does, the lioness or cat and many, many more.

▶ *ToDo*

If you are familiar with a particular goddess tradition, spend some time reacquainting yourself with your favourite goddesses. If you have never met the goddesses before, study the goddess profiles in the Appendix and read as much as you can on the goddesses (local libraries are often fruitful sources of material, see Further Reading). Make a note of any particular traits which you feel could be useful — and of any for which you feel particular antipathy.

Think of someone you particularly dislike. Describe her worst qualities, the things that really get your back up or make you fear her. Is she bossy, matriarchal, judgemental, dominant and controlling, possessive, ambitious for her husband or son? Then she is probably portraying the worst side of Hera, or her equivalent, to you. If she is overly maternal, suffocating, smothering, then Demeter or her equivalent is present. If she is little-girlish, irresponsible, flirtatious, then she is embodying Aphrodite, Persephone or one of the other maiden goddesses. If a goddess does not immediately spring to mind, keep reading until you find just the right one.

Now be very honest with yourself. Are there times when you catch yourself acting like her? Do you have to quell thoughts or actions that would be exactly like hers? Are you afraid that you might turn into her? Take the time to honour and acknowledge that you too have the same qualities; this is your shadow side. Offer her, and yourself, compassion and acceptance (flower essences can be most helpful here).

Look again at her qualities. Then find the quality that is opposite to each of those you dislike so much. This is the hidden potential.

Study someone you admire, envy or wish to emulate. Write down all her 'good' and positive qualities. What does she have that you do not?

Which goddesses are active in her life?

How does she use them?

How do her qualities relate to your own?

How can you integrate these energies positively into yourself? (One way is to identify more strongly with that goddess, see below.)

Identify which of the goddesses' qualities are prominent and which are missing from your life now.

Look back over your life and identify when changes in the goddess energies took place. Is there a goddess who would give you something you feel you lack now? Is one struggling to emerge? If so, how can you help her?

Meeting the Goddesses

Active imagination is a tool to contact the specific energies that the goddesses signify. It is the art of using symbols and images to talk to, and activate, the subconscious part of your mind within which archetypal energy is held. It is a simple technique that requires nothing more than a willingness to let go and see what emerges, and yet it can set in motion constructive change and new experiences.

▶ *ToDo*

Before starting this exercise, choose a goddess who resonates with you or one who has qualities that you wish to make your own.

Read as many different versions of her myth as possible. Study it until you instinctively understand.

If possible, visit a statue of the goddess (most museums have at least one and many of them were magically impregnated with the essence of the goddess as part of the temple rituals).

Find some pictures of the goddess (the *Larousse Encyclopaedia of Mythology* is a useful source). Choose the picture which you feel most epitomises the qualities of the goddess. If possible, stick it in this book.

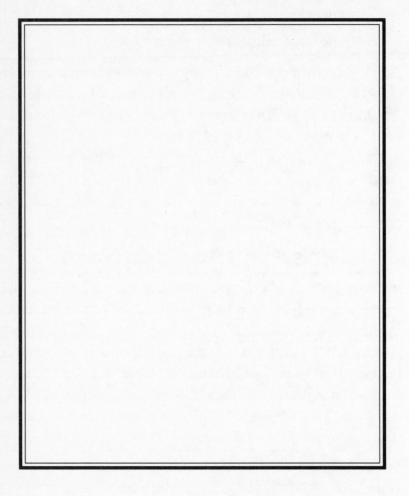

Now sketch or draw your goddess in the space below. The aim is to attune to the energy and to memorise the picture it creates.

Make a list of the things with which your goddess is especially identified. Aphrodite loves roses, for instance. Her colour is pink and her favourite room is the bedroom. She likes beautiful perfumes, sumptuous fabrics and sexy underwear.

Getting to know the goddess

▶ *ToDo*

Choose a quiet time and place where you will not be disturbed and surround yourself with things associated with your goddess. Using the picture you have drawn, or a statue you have chosen, spend a few moments breathing gently and focusing your thoughts on the goddess.

When you are completely relaxed, ask that the goddess will manifest for you. Then, beginning with the head, focus your attention on the image of the goddess until she begins to live for you. Pay special attention to the eyes, looking deep into these and connecting to the being who lives behind them. Slowly work down the figure until you have a living picture in your mind.

At this point close your eyes and concentrate on the inner image, inviting her to manifest her energy within you. Consciously take hold of it as she offers it. Look at life through her eyes. She may take you back to relive her myth, she may take you into an inner experience. Do not be afraid: allow the goddess to reveal to you what you need to know.

When the experience is over, thank her for coming and ask her to be available to you in the future. Then consciously withdraw your attention from the goddess and return it to the everyday world. Be aware of being in your body. Move your hands and feel your feet on the floor. Slowly open your eyes and take time to adjust to being back in the outer world.

Write your experience up in your journal, using the present tense to reinforce it.

This visualisation should be repeated until the goddess is experienced as a living presence. The exercise can then be repeated to contact an energy which is 'missing', or one you are fearful of, or would like to utilise in your life.

Spiritual Sexuality: the Inner Marriage

Every woman is a complex mix of feminine and masculine attributes: passivity and action, receptivity and giving out, birthing and utilising. Accessing, integrating and above all using all your qualities helps you to be a whole person. Having re-membered the parts of your feminine psyche through attunement to the goddesses, it is now time to reintegrate the masculine energies which also form part of your self. This is so no matter what your sexual orientation may be.

This is the alchemical marriage. It can be an important part of your spiritual development as it enables you to reclaim the power normally projected onto a convenient male and gives you access to the 'masculine' qualities of action and initiation. The 'marriage' is within your own instinctual and sacred nature, to the 'god within'. Such an inner marriage is part of the natural progression and cannot be forced. It arises spontaneously in dreams — often through sexual intercourse with a male figure or by phallic symbols (which should be recorded in your journal or painted to make them live). It can be invoked by the use of active imagination.

Although it is possible to tape the exercise, leaving plenty of time to follow the instructions, it is better to memorise it or have someone lead you through it, as this enables you to follow your own inner timing —along with any images which may arise spontaneously as you progress.

Inner marriage medicine

Spiritual Marriage (Findhorn) is especially formulated for making the inner marriage between head and heart, mind and love, will and wisdom, male and female. It brings balance between pairs of opposites, opens the heart to love and intimacy, and brings union and the joy of right relationship.

Tiger Lily (Cal) balances masculine and feminine and integrates them into the psyche.

▶ *ToDo*

▶ **Making the inner marriage**

Choosing a quiet time when you will be undisturbed, sit or lie with your eyes closed. Gently breathe out any tension you may be feeling and breathe in a sense of peace and relaxation. When you are fully relaxed, centre your attention between your eyebrows.

Picture yourself walking up a paved way towards a temple. Feel your feet on the sun-warmed stones. On either side is a row of cypress trees, above you is a clear blue sky. The door to the temple is open. As you enter the temple courtyard, you see that on your left there is a quiet, airy room with a pool. A female attendant waits to bathe and dress you. Enter the water and let it cleanse and purify you.

When she has prepared and perfumed you and dressed you in a clean robe, the attendant gestures to the right side of the temple. Here a temple servant awaits you. He conducts you through the columned arcades of the temple to the offering chamber. Here, on the altar, is the offering you are to make. Offer it up joyfully.

The temple servant then conducts you to the chamber where you will spend the night. The chamber is set for a love feast. Leave your inhibitions at the door as you enter and move towards the sacred marriage bed. Your inner partner awaits you. The love-making is wild and abandoned, tender and gentle, connecting with the primal energies and touching a wellspring of creativity within you. You may even find that you birth a sacred child as a result of this night. Your bridegroom gives you his masculine qualities, enabling you to find them within yourself, to merge and integrate into wholeness.

When you are ready to leave, embrace him and, if possible, let him merge into you. If this is not possible, retain his qualities within yourself. Ask him to be with you when needed. The attendant then conducts you back through the temple to the gateway. As you pass through, the gates close behind you. As you walk back down the paved way, begin to return your awareness to the room. Slowly become aware of your body, of your feet making a firm connection with the earth once again.

When you have completed the visualisation, open your eyes and quietly reflect for a few moments and then record your experience in your journal, or paint a symbolic picture which captures the essence of the union.

Spiritual union with a partner

If you want to find a deeper union with your partner, then you can join on the spiritual level as well as the physical. As this is very powerful, it should only be done with someone you totally and absolutely trust and know you are going to stay with.

▶ *ToDo*

Sit or lie facing each other. (If you wish, you can be sexually joined whilst you carry out this exercise.) Keep your eyes open throughout. Look into each other's eyes.

First of all, synchronise your breathing. Breathe in unison. Breathe right down to your belly: deep, slow breaths. Soon you will feel as though you are being breathed by your partner. Surrender to this feeling.

Then, as you gaze deep into your partner's eyes, connect to the spirit behind the person. Let your own spirit be open to that of your partner. Let the spirits reach out to each other, to merge and join.

Stay like this, looking deep into each other's eyes and breathing together for as long as possible.

It is quite probable that you will find you experience a mutual orgasm, one that takes over your whole body and spirit.

When you have completed, honour the spiritual joining and sharing but know that you must become two people again. Separate from your partner and consciously and deliberately recognise yourself as a separate

*and individual person inhabiting your physical body. See your partner
also as a separate person (this avoids any blurring of boundaries in the
relationship and prevents you giving away your power or taking power
from your partner).*

Soul Retrieval

As you have worked your way through this book, you might have noticed times when you felt lost, empty, joyless, as though a part of you was
missing. You may have noticed that you observe life from the outside.
Your childhood memories may all seem to be from above, as if you were
looking down. You may have identified a curious numbness underlying
depression. You feel as though there is no 'I' present. On the spiritual
level, this may well be so. Whenever you go through trauma, loss, shock
or unbearable pain, or when you are put under strong emotional pressure, then you may suffer what is called 'soul loss'. Soul is the vehicle for
your spirit. So, if you lose part of your soul, your spirit cannot fully
manifest. The spiritual you cannot be fully present in the here and now.

You can also lose soul when your life feels dead, when you give up
your power to others, when you lose sight of yourself. It is as though a
part of yourself leaves, goes to some other place. In shamanic societies
this soul loss has always been recognised as a cause of illness, 'dis-ease'.
The shamans and wise women of the tribe knew how to counteract soul
loss, how to journey to the place of the lost soul, how to bring that soul
back to the body, how to heal the spirit. Serious soul loss can be a
condition that needs the help of an expert. Notwithstanding, the exercises in this book and the contact you have made with the goddesses and
your own inner wisdom will have helped you to counteract any loss of
soul you may have experienced. You can help yourself further through
visualisation and active imagination. You can retrieve your soul.

Note: If you have reason to believe that you were in any way abused
in your childhood, or if you have been through particularly
traumatic events as an adult, then it would be sensible to work with
someone experienced in soul retrieval and healing abuse. (See

Principles of Past Life Therapy, Judy Hall, HarperCollins, London, 1996.) Do not be afraid to ask a prospective therapist if they have experience in the particular aspect of the work you need. If you have a therapist or counsellor, then ask for their cooperation in working with you on the following exercises.

▶ *ToDo*

Look back through your diary and the self-exploration work you have done for this book, and compassionately review your life once again. Does it feel like you, or did it happen to someone else? Can you identify times when you might have suffered from soul loss? Look at the times when you felt dead, disconnected, cut off from life? Notice where you had to give up a part of yourself and what you wanted, in order to stay alive — or to keep the peace. Did you have operations, separations? Did you lose someone you loved? Were you in a car accident? Did you witness anything traumatic? Soul loss can happen even at happy times. Did you give your heart away?

Get out your old photograph albums. Do you always recognise yourself? Do you have a sense that you were present when those photographs were taken? Or were there times when you seem to be elsewhere, somehow missing?

Look at yourself as a child. Were you happy, lively, contented? Or were you rebellious, withdrawn, unhappy? Then look at yourself as a teenager and ask the same questions. Go to your relationships. Did someone take part of you away when he, or she, left? Did you find the man, or woman, of your dreams? And as you grew older did you make your dreams come true, or did they wither and die?

Do you feel complete now? Or is there still a sense of something missing, of inner numbness?

Healing your soul

One of the best healing tools for regaining your soul is forgiveness (see page 162). If you can forgive someone who put you in a situation where you lost your soul, then your spiritual self is alive and well. So, if you have identified someone who may have been involved in the loss of your soul, once you have worked through this, forgive them and let go of the experience. You can only gain by this.

▶ *ToDo*

▶ *Retrieving your lost soul*

Choosing a time and place where you will not be disturbed, settle down and make yourself comfortable. Close your eyes and breathe gently, allowing yourself to relax as deeply as possible. When you are fully relaxed, simply let yourself float up out of your body. You will find that there are threads floating out from you. Each thread is attached to a lost part of your soul. You are going to journey to your own personal place of lost soul. The threads twist themselves into a rope which will guide the way.

The journey starts at the mouth of a cave. There is a long, winding passageway which leads down into the depths. The path has been lighted for you and you will find the rope to guide the way. Follow the rope down the passageway until you come to the place of lost soul.

Here the rope will separate again into threads. Follow each thread to its end, where you will find a piece of your soul. Greet each piece, and ask it to return to you. If it is unsure, ask what it needs to enable it to return. You may need to listen to its story, to hear the tale of how it came to be lost. If so, listen with compassion and love. You may need to offer reassurances, or make promises of change. Be sure that you only make promises you intend to keep. Your soul recognises truth of intention. You may need to reconnect to the you that existed when the piece of soul became lost. To dream again your dreams, to live your hopes and your fears.

As each piece of soul agrees to return, embrace it, welcome it back, take it into yourself. Reabsorb its thread, reconnecting that piece of soul into your inner being. (If a piece of soul is not prepared to return, ask it to wait in this place until you are able to have the help of an expert in soul retrieval.)

When you have followed all the threads, found all the pieces of your soul, and integrated them once more within yourself, then you can begin the journey back. Retrace your steps. Your spirit will instinctively remember the way back.

When you reach the entrance to the cave notice how different you feel, how whole, how vibrant and alive. Remember any promises you have made, any insights you have gained.

Then slowly let yourself settle back into your body. Feel your feet on the ground, the weight of your body in the chair. Breathe a little deeper; move your hands and feet around. When you are ready, open your eyes.

Take time to review what happened and write it up in your journal, using the present tense to anchor and integrate your soul still further.

(If you did find a piece of your soul that was not prepared to return, then seek out a shamanic or soul retrieval practitioner as soon as possible to complete the work.)

Moving On: Cronedom

Now that you have attuned to the archetypal feminine forces with the enormous power they possess and regained the lost parts of yourself, you will experience a tremendous surge of creative energy. This can be put to work for the final stage of growth. This is the moment when everything becomes possible, when the infinite potential open to you can come to fruition. It is time to enter the fourth age of woman: cronedom.

Becoming a crone

First of all, throw away all your notions of what a crone is. She is not an old bag, ugly and withered. Nor is she useless, past her sell-by date. Nor is she a figure of fear — although she has been made to seem that way by those who stand in awe of her power. The crone is the wise woman. The crone is someone who enjoys growing old disgracefully, breaking the taboos of society. She is the grandmother of the tribe, who wears her wrinkles with pride because they come out of experience. Experience that has given her wisdom. Wisdom that entitles her to speak. She wants to be heard, to be honoured. She has much to say, and a great deal that she can teach the young. Recognising the cycles of nature, the crone is unafraid of death. She values life and brings things to birth, but she can also midwife the living through change, endings and dying. Women's wisdom, knowing, insights, skills, spirituality and, above all, that indefinable aura of power are all qualities of cronedom. The crone acts as a guide through the great passages of life. Attuned to the natural cycles and rhythms she is a potent empowerer in maturity.

▶ *ToDo*

▶ *Accessing the crone*

Sit or lie comfortably and close your eyes. Gently breathe out any tension and withdraw your attention into yourself. Take as long as you need to become settled and relaxed.

When you are ready, picture yourself walking down a steeply walled valley. A path will open up in front of you, taking you to the heart of the valley.

At the heart of the valley there is a clearing. At its centre, an old hut. As you reach the hut, a voice will bid you enter. Before you sits an old crone, wrinkled with age. Wise beyond knowing, her bright eyes miss nothing — they peer right through you. She can see into your heart. But she looks with compassion. She too has made this passage. She too has lived her life with all its joys, all its pain.

Spend time with her, ask her to share her wisdom and her experience; learn from her how to reconcile the paradox of opposites; ask her to take you deep within yourself to the place where your knowing resides.

When you are ready to leave, thank her for being there and ask her to be accessible to you whenever you need her.

Then leave the hut and make your way back up the path through the valley, returning to your starting point.

Take deeper breaths and gently return your awareness to the room. Become aware of your surroundings. Take time to adjust and when you are ready open your eyes. Place your feet firmly on the floor and breathe deeply. Write up your experience in your journal.

This visualisation should be repeated from time to time, particularly if the figure was vague or distant at first. It will gradually become easier to access her, and her wisdom.

Crone power

The crone is a powerful woman — which is why she is so often feared and ridiculed by men. Power is one of those words most people fight shy of. Somehow it is seen as something rather nasty, something to be used over people. However, there is another side to power:

Negative power	Positive power
Egocentric	Autonomous
Manipulative	Potent
Exploitative	Impassioned
Power over	Empowering
Destructive	Constructive
Dangerous	Life-enhancing
Devouring	Creative
Uncontrolled	Purposeful
Aggressive	Assertive
Restrictive	Free
Imperative	Discretionary
Covert	Overt
Coercive	Cooperative

You can own your power as a woman and use positive power. You can refuse to take hold of your power, and negative power will be used against you. *The choice is yours.*

▶ *ToDo*

Think about the people you fear, or hold in awe; those who have a hold over you or your life. Who has the most influence in your life now? Who made the rules you live by? You may have to go back into your childhood to see whom you are still obeying, whose view of life you are following (see the Mind section). This is where you meet power issues. Where do you give away your power? To whom? Resolve to take it back!

Recognise your power: Complain, take something unsatisfactory back, boycott, protest, question. As a consumer, you have immense power. Stop buying products that are environmentally unfriendly or hazards to health — and don't be afraid to tell the shop why you are doing this. You do not have to be strident or extreme in order to bring about change; you simply have to stand in your power.

Find a creative project for yourself. Write a book, pass on your skills, teach, talk, paint, run a women's group. Whatever grabs your interest. By now you will know what you are capable of, so take your power in both hands and do it. Now!

Become a crone.

▶ *FactFile*

▶ *Crone medicine*

Wild Woman (DA) brings the freedom to express yourself and creates self-healing.

Rites of Passage

▶ *FactFile*

A rite of passage is a ceremony marking one of the great transition stages in life. It is sacred and honours the moment. It empowers, and brings recognition of the new stage of life. A rite of passage has an inner meaning. It is something private and internal. When viewed from outside, it may merely be the enactment of a drama. Viewed from inside, it is the power of life itself.

Rites of passage have three stages:

1. Withdrawal, isolation, communing
2. The ordeal: a test or symbolic renunciation
3. Renewal, rebirth, re-emergence

▶ *ToDo*

Alone or with a group of friends, create your own rite of passage to mark your menopause. Withdraw from the world, make a retreat. Renounce the past. Be reborn. Celebrate, throw a party, but remember to honour the spirit as well as the body!

The rite of passage below can be done alone or with a group. Working in a peer group reinforces the effect, increases its potency. You can take time for each woman, honouring her and her own unique passage but joining in the sisterhood of women. You may like to ask an older friend who has already passed through menopause to take the part of the crone, the wise woman who guides the ceremony. If so, have her read the instructions out loud. She can then invite each woman in turn to participate.

A rite of passage for menopause

Before you start, gather together everything you will need, including tissues, writing materials, coloured pens, whatever you feel is right. Burn scented candles or incense. Use appropriate background music. Have two tapes: one of sombre, ceremonial music; the other a joyful, uplifting piece. If you have instruments of your own, you may like to play for yourself. Make sure you have a fireplace, or fireproof container, in case you want to burn anything. Dress in bright clothes, covered with a dark cloak or blanket. Dim the lights or simply light a single candle. Play the sombre, ceremonial music quietly.

Settling yourself quietly, withdraw into your cloak. Wrap it around you so that you are dead to the world outside. Go deep down inside. Take time to commune with yourself.

Let your mind go back to the past. To the woman you once were. Acknowledge and honour the feelings attached to the old you in whatever way seems right. You can draw, paint, dance, whatever. Do not be afraid to cry or to feel anger if this is appropriate and stay with the emotion until it passes (if you are allowing yourself to feel the feelings fully, they may well be intense but will not last long). Stay with this phase for as long as feels appropriate.

When you are ready, say out loud:

'I have mourned the past and I now relinquish it and its hold on the present.'

If appropriate, burn anything from the past that you want to let go of. Watch the smoke curling away and allow the past to dissolve. Sit quietly, feeling the burden of the past and all your regrets slipping away. Forgive yourself and anyone else who may have been involved. Let go of the woman you were.

Do not hurry the process but when you have allowed sufficient time for the mourning throw off your cloak to symbolise your new freedom. Let the new you emerge. Honour that new self. Claim the power of the crone. Change the music to something joyous and uplifting. Turn up the lights or light more candles. Look forward with joy and expectation to the new you who has been revealed. If you are working with a group, share with them who you are. State out loud your hopes for the future. Let the others hear and acknowledge you and do the same for them. Wish each other well.

You may like to dance, drum, sing, paint or find some other way to express your joy at who you are. Stay with this feeling for as long as possible, perhaps preparing a celebration meal as a way of ending the rite and carrying the new energy into your everyday life.

And finally,

Make a new life statement.

I am a woman who . . .

Appendix

Goddess Profiles

Feminine wisdom

Sophia

Wisdom, or Sophia, is one of the most ancient concepts. She is the mother, or seed, from which all later wisdom goddesses spring. She is the 'soul of the world', the intuitive face of God. In some of the older myths, she is the Mother of God, existing before all (an idea that passed on into Gnostic Christianity and the Jewish Kabbala). She is a remnant of the Great Goddess who was incorporated into early Judaism. Throughout the Bible we find traces of her peeping out from behind the masculine face of God:

> *Alone, I was fashioned in times long past,*
> *at the beginning, long before earth itself.*
> *When there was yet no ocean I was born.*

— Proverbs 8:22-4

Sophia is a co-creator, the feminine soul of God. Although clearly on the same plane as God, she has independent existence and is actively engaged in relationship with humankind.

She is initiated into the knowledge that belongs to God,
and she decides for Him what He will do.

— Wisdom of Solomon 8

For Sophia herself ranges in search of those who are worthy
of her, on their daily path she appears to them with kindly intent
and in all their purposes meets them halfway.

— Wisdom of Solomon 6:14-17

Sophia is an active principle. The writer of the Wisdom of Solomon chronicles his close and intimate relationship with Sophia. She has sought him out. She was there at his birth, she was the bride he sought. She is the one who has the knowledge of which he would partake. Nevertheless, she is not above testing 'by devious ways' those who would draw close to her. In some versions of her myth, it is Sophia who initiates Adam and Eve into the knowledge of good and evil (although in other interpretations this honour goes to Lilith). In Gnostic Christianity, Sophia is the dove who descends upon Jesus at his baptism bringing to him the spirit of wisdom: the 'holy spirit'. Before she underwent a sex change in the Middle Ages, Sophia was the third member of the Trinity, the Holy Spirit.

Sophia is initiated into the knowledge that belongs to God, and she decides for him what he shall do. According to the Wisdom of Solomon, Sophia knows the past, she can infer what is to come, she understands the subtleties of argument and the solving of problems, she can read signs and portents, and can foretell the outcome of events. These are the attributes of feminine wisdom. Sophia is the archetype of the Wise Woman, feminine wisdom in action, one who epitomises feminine thought. Sophic thought is of a very specific kind. It perceives things as whole, it synthesises and looks at the overall pattern. Sophia's way is logical but empathetic. She combines acute observation with intuitive thought. She takes account of the past in order to project forward into the future. But what Sophia does arises out of care and concern for humankind. Sophic perception uses both the left and right brain modes of thought. It is creative and concerned with vision and solutions.

The negative face of Sophia is closed-mindedness; the fanatic or know-it-all who desperately holds on to what she has been taught as 'right', and who looks down on all those who do not agree with her. She is totally unaware of her own intuitive wisdom, preferring the god of science to the goddess of knowing.

Sophia is the goddess to contact when you need to shift to inward sight so that you can know. Sophia brings you to a point of inner stillness. In the inner stillness you can then listen to her voice bringing you insight and inspiration. She is the source of feminine wisdom.

The Maidens

Aphrodite

Aphrodite's most famous role is that of the beautiful and bountiful goddess of love. The story of her birth, however, illustrates the dark forces which are the other face of love. It is a particularly bloody tale: Cronos castrated his tyrannical father, Uranus, and threw his genitals into the sea. As the sea-foam mixed with the blood, Aphrodite arose fully grown from the waves. Aphrodite quickly became a Greek femme fatale, standing for sexuality and overwhelming libido.

According to legend, Aphrodite had a girdle that made any man vulnerable to seduction, so no man could resist her. Constantly unfaithful to the ugly, lame Hephaistos to whom she was married, Aphrodite was the 'eternal mistress' moving from one steamy affair to the next with god or man as passion took her. Her legendary beauty led to great vanity and in many myths she wrought vengeance on anyone who offended or failed to honour her.

Nevertheless, Aphrodite is also the goddess of music, painting, dance and humour. She is the courtesan, the intelligent, cultured companion. She represents the creative drive, the life force that desires to reproduce itself. As such she is the ideal goddess for any woman wanting to throw off the burden of age, circumstance or marriage, and to know herself as desirable and creative in her own right.

Aphrodite is the archetypal 'love goddess', a woman who epitomises and expresses love on all its levels, and who contains within herself the passion and charisma of the goddess. Aphrodite, however, is an overwhelming urge and many women who are totally attuned to Aphrodite find that they live life driven by a necessity to be desirable, 'feminine'. For such women the menopause, with its intimation of mortality and loss of attractiveness, can be devastating. A woman who is unconsciously acting out the Aphrodite archetype is open to exploitation by men as she desperately seeks assurance of her sexual worth. Such a woman may well find that she attracts misunderstanding from the men she compulsively flirts with, but has little real interest in, and jealousy from the women who look on in condemnation. Other women rarely have much compassion for Aphrodite. They fear her power too much and envy the woman who is freely able to express this archetype.

The Aphrodite shadow is the 'Ice Maiden' whose cold heart is never melted by man. It can be the 'Madonna': sexuality that is deeply repressed, bringing guilt and resentment in its wake. Or the 'Whore': a compulsive acting out of promiscuity that lacks any real contact with the 'lover'. It may be the 'Doormat': an obsessive, dependent relationship in which the woman is constantly humiliated or abused, and yet cannot break free from the chains of 'love'. None of these shadows are able to express the creativity and passion of Aphrodite. They lack her ability to dance lightly through life — although they may themselves break many hearts on their journey. They portray men's 'ideal' even though they do not recognise it within themselves. Recognition is needed before transformation can take place. This transformation is an ability to love oneself and one's innate being.

The positive Aphrodite-woman revels in her sexuality and her sensuality. She lives in and honours her body, but at the same time is capable of channelling all her energy into passionate and spontaneous creations that arise from the breadth of her encompassing imagination.

Athena

Athena is wisdom, a quality believed by the ancient people to be a feminine energy inherent in creation. According to the Greeks Athena sprang fully grown from the head of her father, Zeus, dressed in armour and ready to do battle. Athena is the goddess of wisdom and warriors. She fights alongside the Greek heroes and is a famous strategist. She is also, however, the goddess of crafts and, when not engaged in war, is a patroness of domesticity and creative activities such as weaving.

Living in her head rather than her heart, Athena is one of the great virgin goddesses. Her armour is her defence and protection against sexual entanglements but she nevertheless prefers the company of men with whom she interacts on equal terms.

Athena is a thinking woman. She is rational and logical, good at strategy, a realist. She excels at business, education and political planning. What is more, she is in touch with her femininity so she brings the qualities of compassion and receptivity to bear when making decisions. If the Athena archetype dominates, a woman may be somewhat cold and withdrawn into her intellect but she gives force and direction to what could otherwise be a somewhat passive energy. Where attunement to the archetype is unconscious, she may remain 'Daddy's girl', totally identified with her father and cut off from her mother — for whom she usually has a huge, but unacknowledged, jealousy and rage. A career woman, she lives out all her father's expectations for his girl-child — expectations which centre around success in the masculine world. Academic achievements are highly rated and 'feminine pursuits', which would put her in touch with her inner nature, are spurned. With her father so firmly placed on a pedestal, she is unable to relate to a real flesh-and-blood man either. For this woman, menopause is a confrontation with her unacknowledged self.

The Athena shadow is connected to an urge to live in the head, separated from the body and, in particular, being strongly defended against feelings. Feelings for the Athena shadow are alien territory; she prefers books. The shadow is cold, analytical, passionless and intimidating. Never having been a child, Athena does not know how to play.

Humour and delight are missing from her world. She is thus alienated from her femininity, her core, and needs to attune to the instinctual energies which make her female.

The positive Athena-woman is able to make choices based on compassionate reason, rather than on emotion, and yet at the same time is rooted in her femininity. Attuning to Athena at the midlife transition can enable a woman to plan her future, to move beyond the instinctual child-rearing years, putting her skills to work in the larger world.

Artemis

Artemis is goddess of the moon, the hunt and childbirth. An instinctual nature-goddess of the waxing moon, she was worshipped as the mother goddess for thousands of years before the patriarchal gods of classical Greece came into being. Nevertheless, she was, as were so many others, incorporated into the myths as yet another child of Zeus. This time, however, Artemis was born out of one of Zeus's seductions and the myths show her mother Leto, a nature deity, in conflict with Hera (Zeus's wife) who cursed her. Owing to Hera's wrath, Leto had great difficulty in finding anywhere to give birth, eventually ending up on the sacred but barren island of Delos. Her daughter Artemis was born quickly and without pain, but her labour continued agonisingly for many days until eventually Artemis was able to help birth her twin, Apollo. Artemis was always close to her brother, a sensitive, music-loving being, and he features strongly in her myth. She was also extremely protective of her mother (unusual in the Greek myths) and she could be seen as aiding her mother to birth her own masculine side — that is, to bring it into consciousness.

When the twins were three, Leto took them to Olympus to meet their father. Zeus was charmed by the small girl and offered to give her all she desired. She asked for a short tunic, bow and arrows, a pack of hounds, and the mountains and wild places as her very own. Finally, she asked for nymphs as companions and eternal chastity, so Artemis is yet another of the virgin goddesses. However, in her myths she makes love to her nymphs, so Artemis is also the lesbian goddess who explores feminist sexuality.

Artemis is a shaman who understands the link between instinct and magic. She is the woman with an instinctual attunement to nature and the wild places, who needs freedom. Artemis spent her days hunting with her friends; sometimes returning to lead the evening dancing; but she hung her own quiver outside her hut to fool men into believing she had a lover there. Artemis has forsworn men, and she has the qualities of independence and one-with-herselfness with which many lesbians can easily identify but which are also appropriate to all women at midlife, no matter what their sexual orientation may be.

Artemis is whole, intact, independent and free-spirited. At ease with and able to express the masculine part of her nature, she knows what she wants and where she is going. Some women may be stuck in the phase of the archetype which is perennially adolescent, refusing to move into the sexual fullness of womanhood; or may be living out the archetype through dependent lesbian relationships rather than becoming whole within themselves. The archetype may well suddenly appear in middle-age, calling a woman to leave her home and family and seek out the wild places in herself, perhaps through relationship with another woman, or through shamanism or wicca.

The Artemis shadow is restless, always on the move, the huntress who brings pain and suffering to her victims (many of the myths tell of the pain inflicted by this dual goddess). Conversely, she may be pliant, dependent, desperately afraid to find her own independent self. She may be the militant, man-hating feminist who wants to ban men from the planet or who blames them for all the troubles of the world.

The positive Artemis-woman is, however, a midwife for the planet and a fitting archetype for the wise-woman phase. It is she who will bring through the ancient knowledge inherent in her dance. This knowledge is that the Earth and all upon it are sacred, intact, at-one; brothers and sisters all; interplaying in the eternal, instinctual rhythm symbolised by this ancient moon goddess. She is midwife for the sacred nature, here to teach that we are spiritual beings on a human journey. For anyone entering fearfully on the midlife rite of passage, Artemis is the ideal companion: protective, skilled and instinctual, she can lead a woman into the centre of her own being.

The Matrons

Hera

Hera is power. The wife of the head of the Greek pantheon, Zeus, and the goddess of marriage, her own marriage appears to have been far from happy. Zeus was the arch-philanderer. The Greek myths are full of his adultery and resulting offspring — and Hera's legendary jealousy and rage. According to myth, poor Hera did not have a happy childhood. She was a child of Rhea and Cronos, swallowed by her father as she was born. She was liberated when her brother Zeus forced his father to disgorge his children. In her early life she may have been overshadowed by her father, but Hera was not a weak woman. When Zeus tried to seduce her, she failed to succumb and forced him to marry her. The honeymoon is said to have lasted for 300 years. Even though the two of them carried on a 'war of the sexes', Hera was nevertheless powerful. Zeus was afraid of offending her too much for fear of what she would do in retaliation, and she had her own secret rites which hint at a deeper power. She was able to self-create and birth the terrible Typhon, a scourge of humankind.

One Hera-woman is the Wife, a paragon of domestic virtue. She yearns for the prestige and status that marriage, in her eyes, confers. Within the home, she is 'she who must be obeyed', the dominant matriarch and the backbone of many charitable institutions. Like Hera before her, she will put up with a great deal in order to retain her position — even to the extent of turning a blind eye to her husband's infidelity or addiction, so long as she remains 'the Wife'. When she is aware of the affair, she blames the other woman, not her husband. She is the 'power behind the throne', supporting and urging her husband ever onward and upward on the power ladder. And yet the Hera-woman is jealous of his power and his mobility, which she wants for herself but may not know how to get.

In the Hera Career Woman, who has made her way in the world, the male side dominates. This is the woman who lives out all that her father most wanted in a son. She must be that son, must succeed at all costs. She has no time for 'feminine things'. Ruthless, confident, arrogant and her father's daughter, her sterile creations may well become the scourge of the world.

The Hera shadow is the jealousy, possessiveness and vindictive temper which Hera could display only too well. But this is based on her inner feeling of powerlessness, of incompletion unless she has a mate, and her fear of loss of self that would result if she were alone. Many of the strident feminists who sought to replace men were reflecting the Hera shadow, as are the highly successful man-gutting businesswomen and female politicians who strive to dominate their world. Unconscious attunement to the Hera archetype may equate with refusing the midlife rite of passage that would link what a woman has been with what she may be. Part of the Hera shadow may be a reluctance to move forward, to change or to grow; trying instead to cling to the past and 'how it was'. Such a woman cannot face up to the loneliness, and the challenge, of developing a sense of independent self.

Society has singularly failed the Hera wife. Her values are no longer the norm, her security is at risk, and her power, which she so needs to own, is not valued. The lack of a socially defined role for the older woman strikes most lethally at the heart of the Hera-woman. She is the one who most misses a rite of passage which would validate her existence, the woman who most needs a sense of continuity to unite past and future so that they meet in the present.

Hera's strongest quality is commitment and her greatest potential is to own her power and become a woman in her own right.

Hestia

Hestia is the goddess of the hearth. The elder sister of Hera and Zeus, she shared the fate of being swallowed by her father but, unlike Hera, when disgorged she actively reclaimed power over her life and refused to hand it over again. Having declined the courtship of both Poseidon and

Apollo, she chose instead to remain a virgin and tend the fire at the heart of every home.

She took little part in Olympian mythological life, but was much venerated by the Greeks as her sacred fire made any place holy (that is, the spirit of the god or goddess dwelt there). Hestia was linked to the Vestal Virgins in Rome who tended the sacred flame. At around the age of forty the virgin priestesses had to make the choice of whether to remain in the temple and instruct the younger priestesses, or to go out into the world again and carry their spirituality with them: so there is a strong connection between Hestia and the midlife transition.

Hestia is virgin, intact. She does not need a man to make her complete, although she may choose to share her life with one or with someone of her own sex. She is the wise woman with an inward-seeing eye and a quiet tranquillity that nothing disturbs. She represents harmony and order and is present in the woman who enjoys her work for the sake of the task itself: being present in the moment. Hestia is the personal assistant who quietly and efficiently supports her boss; the nurse who carries out her tasks with compassion and caring; the nun who devotes her life to the young; the worker amongst the down-and-outs. The Hestia-woman is far more likely to be quietly pursuing the spiritual pathway than climbing the career ladder. In Hestia-women in whom devotion to matters of the spirit has been outwardly unapparent for the first half of life, a change will come about at the midlife point and their spiritual leanings will become more defined and urgent.

Detachment is one of Hestia's qualities and this may lead to the shadow of a woman who appears unaware of the needs of others, seemingly cold and uncaring because of her inwardly focused self. It may also lead to the 'wishy-washy' type of 'spiritual woman', commonly found in ashrams and communities, whose attention is so inwardly focused that she is incapable of managing out in the world. Or to the celibate who has renounced sexuality, finding virtue in repression, and who equates 'virgin' with untouchable rather than the old meaning of intact and whole. The Hestia shadow can also be present in the woman who 'serves others' from a sense of no-self, a lack of inner value and worth; or from a sense of moral superiority and a kind of inverted snobbery; or the 'religious' woman who serves the letter of the law rather than its intent and who imposes her own morality and judgement on others in the certainty that she knows what is good for them.

Not attached to people or outcome, the positive Hestia-woman is centred in herself and offers a wise perspective from which to view the world. In her role of keeper of the hearth, she is the centre that nourishes others from her resource of spiritual power. She has inner light and a strong connection to her self which gives her the potential to be a truly Wise Woman.

Maiden and Mother

Persephone and Demeter

Demeter is the corn goddess, the earth-mother, and her story is the myth of the triple aspects of creation: conception, preservation and destruction — the cycle of life. It is also a story of letting go and of reconciliation, the archetypal mother and daughter tale. When we meet Demeter, she is Mother and her maiden aspect is personified by her daughter, Kore or Persephone. Demeter was one of the many sister-wives of Zeus and she shared the fate of her sisters in that she was swallowed by her father for part of her young life. She is also one of the goddesses who gives birth to a son that becomes her consort, although she is perhaps best known as the archetypal 'one-parent family' in the role of mother of Persephone. It is this aspect on which her myth centres. Persephone is, naturally enough, a beautiful maiden who is desired by Pluto (Hades), god of the Underworld. He connives with Zeus, the girl's father, to arrange her abduction. One moment Persephone is innocently picking flowers with her companions. The next, as she puts out her hand to a particularly beautiful flower, the earth opens up beneath her feet and Pluto emerges in his chariot, snatches her up and takes her to his kingdom — Hades, the abode of the dead.

Demeter, who has heard Persephone's cries, searches frantically for nine days for her lost daughter. Her grief is so great that she does not eat, sleep or bathe. On the tenth day she meets the third face of woman, the waning-moon goddess Hecate. Hecate takes her to Helios, a sun god, who tells Demeter of the plot to kidnap her daughter and points out Zeus's part in the matter. Helios suggests that she should accept the situation. Demeter, however, refuses to accept the betrayal by her own brother. She retires from Olympus and, disguised as an old woman, wanders the countryside until she is given a job as a nursemaid. Here, in parallel with the Egyptian Isis myth, she begins to make the child divine. Each night she holds him in a fire to make him immortal. Unfortunately, as with Isis, the child's mother intervenes to stop the process.

Demeter reveals her true identity and has a temple built for her in which she sits and grieves for her child. This is a serious matter, as Demeter is goddess of the corn and without her nothing will grow. Finally Zeus sends messengers to her imploring her to return. But, furious still, Demeter refuses until her daughter is returned to her. Hermes, messenger of the gods, is sent to Hades where he seemingly finds a depressed and weepy Persephone only too eager to return to her mother. Pluto agrees to return her, but first he gives her pomegranate seeds to eat. Had she not accepted the pomegranate seeds, Persephone could have returned to life above ground permanently. As it is, she has tasted the fruit of knowledge and she must spend a period of the year below ground with Pluto as Queen of the Underworld.

The Demeter myth contains many vignettes, one of which is the child who is to be made divine. It is an allegory for the psychological dissolution which splits off the child who is within every woman, who must be purged and purified by fire in order to reveal the goddess within. Unfortunately, most mothers (that is woman herself) are afraid for the child and refuse to let it go through the ordeal which will bring immortal life. Demeter, like her Egyptian sister Isis, as the great mother who has known loss, can facilitate this process of dissolution, purification and reunification with the divine force.

Demeter is the archetypal mother and nurturer. She is the maternal instinct personified and it is the Demeter archetype who suffers from the 'empty nest syndrome' simply because her instinct to have children is so strong and her grief at the loss of her fertility so overwhelming. Her nourishment is not only for her children, however. Demeter provides physical, psychological and spiritual nurture for all — particularly in the 'helping professions'. Nevertheless, she also encompasses the opposite principle. When the goddess's child is taken away, she rages and cuts off support for humankind. The earth becomes barren.

When the Demeter-woman's 'child' leaves home, she may well fall into deep depression and see this as 'the end', no matter what other responsibilities she may have. Her response to loss, or threat, is to withhold nurturing; to refuse to meet the needs of others or of herself. So the Demeter-woman's reaction to midlife may well be to withdraw, to be unavailable. Her children, for instance, who have made lives for themselves may find that they are approved of only if that life fits into what mother 'knows' will be right for them. Her husband may find that he has lost his wife while she struggles to let go of her children, or her desire to have children. Demeter-women often see themselves as victims; they give until literally they have nothing left to give and then deeply resent the calls made on their exhausted energies. Above all else Demeter needs to learn how to say 'No'; to make choices rather than to be compelled to nurture.

The Demeter shadow is possessiveness allied to fear of loss, purposelessness and depression. It is 'passive-aggression', hostility that is hidden and fearful, based on unspoken resentment and unacknowledged feelings. It 'forgets to do' rather than saying a clear no. Demeter is afraid of the Underworld (i.e. the unconscious) and refuses to allow her daughter to go through the psychological integration that exploring the depths of the psyche can bring. The Demeter shadow, therefore, may prefer to 'help' someone, thereby keeping them dependent, rather than allow them to explore their own shadow and become whole once more. It can also be an exploitative shadow, manipulating and manoeuvring to get its own way. It is the 'little girl' who refuses to grow up, the woman who calls her husband 'daddy', and especially the woman who refuses to make the transition to the 'crone' or wise woman aspect of life. This shadow is the mother who has to be nurtured by her children, who must be placated and wooed for fear she turns into the devouring mother. Her unspoken threat is loss of love.

The positive Demeter-woman, on the other hand, has faced loss and come through with increased wisdom so she can accompany others on their journey. She has learnt how to mother herself, to be her own child, with love and generosity but also with a protective awareness that allows her to know when enough is enough (both for herself and others). She has an attunement to the cycles of nature. She understands the need for death. She knows how to be in the dark place where new seeds sprout. She does not constantly poke around to be sure they have germinated, which would snuff them out. She is content to wait for everything to mature in its season, knowing that the harvest will come.

Persephone has two faces. Her 'young' face is the maiden, Kore, who was an integral part of the fertility trinity. Her much more ancient face is the mature goddess, the Queen of the Underworld, who rules over dead souls and guides the living who wish to journey there. Nor is she an innocent, faithful to her husband. In at least one myth she fights with Aphrodite over the beautiful Adonis (who, ironically, had been sent to her for safe-keeping). This myth is an allegory involving the consort who dies and rises again. Whilst in Persephone's keeping he is dead, but returned to Aphrodite, goddess of love, he is life itself and the return of fertility.

If a woman is attuned to the Kore archetype, she is ever-youthful, sexually unawakened and uncommitted. She is often totally dependent on her mother, and frequently acts out the part of 'anima-woman' for men. Pliable and unformed, she is seemingly all things to all men because she reflects what they wish to see, she who delights in pleasing. Clearly this characteristic can also form part of the Persephone shadow. A singular naivety and insularity can lie at the heart of the apparently lustful woman. She finds her own unawakened sexuality and lack of commitment reflected back to her in the men who, in her unseeing eyes, reject her desire for closeness and union. Such a woman may, either actually or metaphorically, find herself living the abduction and rape of Persephone when Pluto bursts through from the underworld: potentially as a crisis which activates and moves her into the mature Persephone role, although it may merely be a repetitive pattern.

'Unawakened' Persephone, powerless and passive, is the 'eternal, sacrificial victim'. She projects all her power out there onto mother, matriarch or man. She eternally re-creates the conditions which lead to her downfall. Such a maiden desperately needs to be handed over to the dark powers for a journey down into her own unconscious, so that those powers can be made sacred and integrated through an initiation of the mature spirit. She is then the reconciliation of the opposites of dark and light — the integration of the powerful, unconscious forces of the psyche with the brightness of consciousness.

When the mature, receptive Persephone archetype is activated, this is the guide to the underworld: the woman who is at home in the realm of the intuition and the unconscious; one who has the capacity for deeply moving spiritual and sexual experiences which take her beyond herself to unity with the cosmos. She is psychic and perceptive, attuned to forces beyond the comprehension of most women; and is the potential midwife for birthing the sacred nature in everyone.

Mature Persephone can be most helpful for women who have undergone any kind of abuse. Mature Persephone has regained her power, has overcome her abduction and violation, and has found healing in the darkness. The positive Persephone-woman is at home within the depths of the psyche, and can act as a guide for others journeying into their own unconscious. She is attuned to the birth-death-rebirth cycle and may find herself instinctively drawn to work with the dying, aiding them not only in their transition to another life but also showing them how to live fully until they die.

Crone

Hecate

Hecate is the ancient lunar goddess of the crossroads, the all-seeing eye who looks in three directions at once; ruling heaven, earth and the underworld. She is an ancient divinity associated with magic and prophecy but metamorphosed into one of Hera's children. In a myth, she incurred the wrath of her mother (by stealing Hera's rouge) and hid in the bed of a woman who was giving birth. The contact with the puerperal blood rendered Hecate impure and she was plunged into the Acheron (one of the rivers leading to Hades) to be cleansed. As a result she became a goddess of the Underworld.

As the goddess of enchantment and magic, Hecate is linked to choices and to the Way. She is at her most powerful when the Moon wanes, the instinctual time. She rules the great crossroads of a woman's life, such as puberty, marriage and menopause when this power is closest to the surface. She has a torch to light the darkness and thus performs the function of taking one deep into oneself, and of linking the conscious mind with the unconscious. She is therefore an excellent guide for inner work. She is also a goddess of purification who presides at initiations and rituals. She witnessed the abduction of Persephone, and was able to act as mediator when Demeter tried to rescue her daughter; thus she has the function of bringing together lost parts of the self. Indeed, Hecate can be seen to be presiding over Persephone's initiation and descent into the unconscious, accompanying her return and spiritual illumination. In Hecate we have the completion of the trinity: the Crone is united with Mother and Maiden.

The Hecate-woman is the link between the different levels of consciousness and can move between them with confidence. She understands the magical dimension of life. Not afraid to face death and old age, she is unlikely to withhold her power for fear of men — over whom she may well hold a dark enchantment. She is the Morgan le Fay of the Arthurian legends, a woman who fascinates men with her aura of mystery and magic and the threat of her power.

The Hecate shadow may well be linked to this fascination, and to dark powers used unconsciously to manipulate and coerce those around her. Her link to the depths is great, but her awareness is shallow, and therefore everything dark and mysterious is projected onto 'another'. Thus, in the outer world the Hecate shadow will constantly encounter that which she avoids owning in herself: power. When the Hecate-woman does not consciously own her power, and thereby use it wisely, she may well take others down into the darkness but deny responsibility, ensuring their disintegration.

The positive Hecate archetype is extremely helpful for those making the midlife rite of passage. As Crone, Hecate lights the way and shares her sacred wisdom. Hecate is the third age of woman. When the Hecate-woman consciously integrates her shadow and owns her power, she can act as a light for those who are penetrating their own darkness and can bring together the lost parts of the self.

Mother, Wife and Wise Woman

Isis

Isis is the archetypal devoted wife and mother — pictorial representations show her nursing her son, Horus, in a madonna-and-child-like pose — but Isis is much more than this. She was one of the goddesses of power in whose honour a great mystery was re-enacted each year: that of death and resurrection. She utilised magic when necessary, and the power of life and death was an integral part of her myth — she brings Osiris back to life and treats her son for a fatal scorpion bite — and of her worship. The initiation rites of Isis included a symbolic death and return to the grave, from which the initiate would arise reborn. Her great festival celebrated the annual fertility-bearing inundation of the Nile. She is one of the great embodiments of the core belief of the Egyptians: life after death. Isis and Osiris are part of the great cycle of birth, death and rebirth. Isis is one of the goddesses who has the psychological function of uniting lost parts of the self, as her myth shows.

Osiris, Isis's consort, had a brother, Seth. Seth, an ancient Upper-Egyptian god who in the earliest myths assisted the dead, became a dark twin and, in the later myths, the personification of evil. He is associated with natural phenomena that shut out the light of the sun, such as clouds, storms, earthquakes, darkness and, most terrifying of all for ancient peoples, eclipses. Thus, Osiris and Seth fragment and polarise the opposites of good and evil, day and night, light and dark, life and death, which Isis ultimately reconciles.

According to the Osiris myth, Seth became envious of his brother and desired to take over power for himself. Seth had a richly decorated chest carefully constructed and then gave a feast for Osiris. At the height of the feast, the chest was carried in and Seth promised to give it to the man it would fit. Although many tried, no one could fill the stature of the king and eventually he was persuaded to try the box. No sooner had he lain down than conspirators slammed the lid and nailed it shut. The chest was then thrown into the Nile.

Isis, an intuitive psychic, knew immediately of her husband's assassination and went into mourning. Full of grief, she set off to seek the chest. Whilst on this journey she was told that Nephthys, her sister and wife of Seth, had been seduced by Osiris and had borne him a son. Nephthys, terrified of what Seth might do, had exposed the child immediately after birth but the child had been saved by wild dogs. Isis located the pack of dogs and rescued her nephew, whom she named Anubis. She forgave her sister, who left her husband and joined Isis in the hunt for Osiris.

News reached the sisters that the chest had been washed ashore at Byblos and Isis went there to search for it. It had been thrown into the branches of a tamarisk tree, which grew around the chest and encompassed it into its trunk. This tree became famous for its wonderful size and beautiful flowers, and the local king had it cut down to make a pillar for his palace. When Isis arrived, she simply sat without speaking and the handmaidens of the queen, intrigued by the beautiful stranger, engaged her in conversation. Isis showed them how to braid their hair and make themselves beautiful, covering them in a sensuous fragrance. When the queen heard of the beautiful stranger, she herself went to welcome her.

The queen's child was ill and Isis offered to heal him. Each day she would shut the queen out and place the child in flames to burn away his mortality. Unfortunately the queen was unable to resist interfering, but she recognised Isis as a goddess and the child became well. As a reward, Isis asked for the pillar that contained Osiris's body. She split open the tree, removed the chest and returned the pillar to the king and queen. She then began to lament for her lost lord, and so terrifying was her grief that one of the queen's sons died of fright.

Isis loaded the chest onto a ship and returned to Egypt, where she immediately set about reviving Osiris. A beautiful Egyptian verse tells of her magic, which was able to warm and breathe life into Osiris's body long enough for it to impregnate her with her son, Horus. Seth returns to the story and imprisons Isis, but she escapes and attempts to give birth alone, in the reeds. The birth, however, is a difficult one and ultimately two gods arrive, mark Isis with a cross of blood — the sign of life — and her son is born. Horus is destined to become the new solar lord, taking over from the old solar god, Ra. This birth takes place at the vernal equinox, the first day of Spring, when the young corn sprouts. Isis continues to be hunted by Seth and many misfortunes befall her whilst her son is little. She is a goddess who has lost everything including divine protection and has to fall back on her own power.

Seth continues to be active in the story. This time he finds the chest with Osiris's body and cuts it into fourteen pieces, which he flings into the Nile. Isis sets off again in search of her husband and, after many trials and tribulations, she finds the missing pieces. Each time she finds a piece, she apparently buries it and builds a shrine, although this is a trick to fool Seth. Only one piece is missing, the phallus of Osiris which has been eaten by a fish. So, when she reassembles the body, it has a wooden phallus. Horus meanwhile has done battle with his evil uncle and vanquished him. Horus then takes his uncle's eye to where Isis waits with Osiris's body. He opens his father's mouth and gives him the eye to eat (symbol of eternal life). Osiris is then able to ascend his shaman's ladder to 'heaven' where, in the afterlife, it becomes his task to judge the lives of mortals, and it is Osiris and his son Anubis who meet them at the entrance to the otherworld.

Isis, therefore, is that part of the great goddess who marries only to lose her consort to the forces of nature (the birth-death-rebirth cycle) but who retains the power of regeneration. She is unconditional love, as shown by her forgiveness of her sister; a goddess of courage, who endures long after she has lost everything; and one who understands grief and its part in the creative process of life. In persevering with her search for the scattered parts of Osiris, she re-members her own male side.

In an interesting piece of symbolism, Isis teaches the handmaidens to braid their hair and make themselves beautiful. Hair has long been a symbol for wisdom — and for seduction. Here Isis is helping the maidens attune to their essential feminine nature. She is teaching them the rituals of adornment, rituals that can lead a woman into a deeper knowledge of her inner nature.

Isis is a useful goddess, then, for a woman who wants to contact her feminine self, one who needs to make the sacred marriage or to birth her own divine child. She is also helpful, as is Demeter, where a woman is entrenched in a 'loss' phase of life. Isis knew when to let go, to allow Osiris to go with the natural flow and return to the otherworld from whence he came. Attuning to Isis can, therefore, aid the woman who has lost her partner or her role in life, or who is simply mourning the loss of her fertility.

Isis is a goddess of initiation and her initiates were given a many-coloured veil which represented the varied forms of nature in which the all-present spirit is clothed. Putting on the veil of Isis can allow a woman to attune to the incarnation of spirit into matter, to reunion with her own spirituality so that she becomes virgin, intact and sacred once more.

Devourer and Healer

Sekhmet

Sekhmet is the dark, destroying face of the goddess. Sekhmet is usually depicted as a lion-headed woman and Hathor, the light face of the goddess, as a cow or as a beautiful woman wearing cow's horns. Hathor was the patroness of women and the goddess of love, music and dancing: her rituals featured musical instruments and dancing girls, and her temples were 'places of intoxication'. In a beautiful little temple at Philae the gods are depicted as animals playing and dancing with great joy and abandon at one of Hathor's festivals.

This is in stark contrast to the statues and representations of Sekhmet who is almost always shown in her awesome aspect. The best-known legend about Sekhmet features her as the avenging 'Eye of Ra'. In his declining years Ra was mocked by his 'subjects', the Egyptians. Angry, he plotted revenge. Sekhmet, in the form of a rampaging lioness, was sent forth to destroy humankind and quickly discovered a delight in killing. Her blood lust could not be satiated and she killed everyone she met. Ra, feeling that his vengeance had been completed, asked her to stop but Sekhmet, who had divine power and could overrule even Ra, would not be halted. The Nile and the land of Egypt ran red with blood.

Ra sent his messengers to Elephantine Island, at Aswan in Upper Egypt, to gather the fruit of the mandrake, the juice of which is blood-red and has a powerful sedative effect. Women brewed seventy thousand gallons of beer, mixed it with the mandrake juice and poured it out on the earth to form a lake of blood. When Sekhmet passed by, she drank the lethal brew and went quietly to sleep. When she awoke, Thoth, the baboon god of wisdom, led her home in peace, telling her humorous tales to help her forget her hangover. Obviously a transformation took place, as from then on she is depicted as a healer goddess, one who watches over initiation and childbirth. Thoth is the personification of wisdom in Egyptian mythology. The myth of Sekhmet can, therefore, be seen as the growth of wisdom; the conquering, or sublimation, of the instinctual side of life and the flowering of the spiritual element.

Sekhmet is the goddess to contact when courage is needed: 'the strength of a lion', when action has to be taken, when something has to die, when transformation is called for, or the reconciliation of opposites undertaken. If a woman is in the grip of an overwhelming instinct such as self-destruction or is suddenly desperate for another child, then contacting Sekhmet will help her to attune to the positive benefit of that archetype: destroying the old so that the new can arise, for instance, or creating from the non-biological level. As Sekhmet understands betrayal and humiliation, she is a goddess to contact for healing old abuse of any description. Like so many of the goddesses, she also has the power to take you deep within yourself, to meet your shadow, and to birth the sacred self.

Power

Kali

Kali was born from the ocean of blood at the beginning and end of the world, the symbolic flux from which all is created and to which all returns. She is Time, the cycle of creation. The Indian sage Ramakrishna described her as 'the dark formlessness of pre-creation chaos' and 'the shining ocean of consciousness'. She is past, present and future. Power is an integral part of Kali — one of her many names is Shakti, or power. This power is creative, maintaining and destroying: 'The whole Universe rests upon Her, rises out of Her and melts away into Her.' She is the triple-faced goddess of creation, preservation and destruction, who is best known in her function of devouring mother epitomising the terrible, indissoluble link between birth and death, womb and tomb. Kali is, however, also 'Mother of all living' and the 'Treasure-House of Compassion (Karuna), Giver of Life'. She is the fount of all love that flows through the world, and women are believed to be her flesh made mortal. In one of her aspects she is the beautiful goddess Durga (paradoxically, a great slayer of demons), in another the black earth-mother and in yet another the harvest bride.

Kali is usually depicted in her 'hideous' aspect. In one form she is shown standing grinning on the prostrate form of her partner Shiva, with an outstretched tongue. Her body is smeared in blood because she has waged a ferocious battle. Around her neck is a necklace of skulls. She has four arms, one of which holds a weapon, another a head dripping blood, with the other two held out in blessing. Another more graphic form shows her squatting over the corpse of Shiva, her consort, drinking his blood while her yoni (vagina) devours his phallus. In one myth Kali is sent out to destroy. As with Sekhmet, she rejoices in the slaughter and will not stop. When Shiva approaches her and lies down among her victims, Kali leaps on to him. In shame, she ejects her tongue. However, in the Tantric version, Kali is actually rejuvenating Shiva with her magical, potent menstrual flow and her tongue is extended in an expression of sexual ecstasy.

Kali is, therefore, another of the great goddess forms who aids in transformation, who devours what is old and outworn but provides the regenerative energy for new creation. She can integrate masculine and feminine within herself. A woman who can make a friend of Kali in her terrifying aspect need never again be afraid of death — or anything else for that matter. She will learn that life and death form an indissoluble, creative bond, and that one cannot exist without the other.

Primal Woman

Lilith

So God created man in his own image; in the image of God he created them; male and female he created them.

And so the Lord God put the man into a trance, and while he slept, he took one of his ribs and closed the flesh over the place. The Lord God then built up the rib, which he had taken out of the man, into a woman.[7]

Have you ever wondered why there are two versions of the creation story in the Bible? In one, man and woman are created equal and at the same time (on the fifth day). In the other, woman is created from man, leading to dependency and inferiority. Well, Lilith is the answer. She fits neatly into the gap between 'the creation of the world' and 'the beginnings of history' and, although she no longer features in the Bible, she is recorded in Hebrew legend and flies through Middle Eastern mythology as a goddess of the night. Lilith was Adam's first consort and very different from the pliable Eve. Sinuous and sensual, she was 'the winding serpent' and was portrayed as winged and part snake (you will of course recall that it was a serpent who later tempted Eve in the garden).

Adam means 'son of the red Mother Earth' and in the earliest creation stories it was a Mother Goddess who was responsible for creation, so the Adamic creation story incorporates a much earlier, matriarchal legend which has become patriarchal. All the elements of goddess worship appear in the biblical story: the cosmic serpent, the garden, the Tree of Life with its fruit of knowledge, and the sexual rites which lead to illumination. Hebrew legend tells us that Adam married Lilith because he was tired of coupling with the beasts.

Lilith is reputed to have left Adam because he insisted on the missionary position, symbolic of the male dominance he wished to establish, and to which Lilith refused to acquiesce. Rebellious and autonomous, having cursed him she flew away to live by the Red Sea. When God sent the angels to fetch her back, she cursed them too. She then spent her time 'coupling with demons', allegedly producing up to one hundred children a day: the 'Lilim' (night hags or harlots of hell) who featured strongly in medieval religious horror tales. Lilith and her offspring appear throughout the Bible and Jewish mythology, always placing man's soul in mortal danger. She is 'the part of the feminine that is experienced as seductive witch, outcast and shadow'. According to the Jews of the Middle Ages and the Christian clerics of the time, the Lilim caused wet dreams, laughing whenever a pious Christian was so afflicted. After an encounter with a night hag (a beautiful creature despite her name), mortal man would never again be satisfied with a mortal woman. Monks are reputed to have slept with their hands crossed over their genitals to fend off the night hag, the seductive advances of the dark goddess who flies in the darkness.

Lilith is another of the dual goddesses, whose powers are most fearful at the waning moon, activating the dark side of the Goddess whom men have feared for millennia. She 'personifies the neglected and rejected aspects of the Goddess'. In the Hebrew myths she is seductive woman, beautifully adorned; beguiling, fascinating and totally irresistible. With her long dark hair she is wisdom personified, but that wisdom is feared and forbidden by man. Meeting Lilith at the ritual of her adornment can lead a woman into a far deeper awareness of her own awesome powers and a psychological integration with the real nature of femaleness which has been shut off for so long.

In legend Lilith is portrayed as a child killer, equating perhaps to those mythological mothers who would kill the 'children of their imagination' rather than risk 'their own individuality and passion'. She is creativity itself and nothing is allowed to stand in her way. And, as Barbara Black Koltuv points out, her 'child-killing' equates to freedom from our own childish aspect that needs love and approval from others in order to be able to function. So Lilith is a goddess for a woman seeking the instinctual side of femininity who wants to honour and integrate the dark aspect of the Goddess. She is the model for a woman who is looking for strength and independence and the ability to say 'No' whether seeking sexuality or liberation. Lilith sought freedom rather than bondage. She is the quality in woman that will not submerge itself in a relationship but rather demands true equality, and the freedom to change and grow into her total self.

Lilith understands rejection but accepts herself. She is original woman, virgin in the sense of being whole and intact; sexually liberated, fertile, fecund and creative — a creature who lives by the Red Sea, the sea of blood which features strongly in the legends of her fellow ancients Sekhmet and Kali and which is 'the material substance of generation' (Pliny).

Resources

NATURAL HORMONE SUPPLIERS

The Natural Health Ministry
Well-Woman Nutrition Centre
Mcintyre, Donegal Town
County Donegal
IRELAND
Tel: Advice Line: 01648 44444

NATURAL HORMONES AND NUTRITIONAL
SUPPLEMENTS

Youthinol, Orachel:
Neways International UK Ltd.
Allison & Tom Kelly
Harvard Way
Kimbolton, Huntingdon
Cambridge PE18 0NY
Tel: 01480 86174

Wild Yam cream:
Primavera Aromatherapy Preparations Ltd
Mells, Frome, Somerset BA11 3QZ, UK
Order Line: 01737 813678

Natural Progesterone Information Service
BCM Box 4315, London WC1N 3XX, UK

FLOWER ESSENCE SUPPLIERS:

The Working Tree
Milland, Liphook, Hants GU30 7JS, UK
Tel: 01428 741572

Petaltone Essences
David Eastoe
6 Behind Berry, Somerton, Somerset, UK

Green Man Tree Essences
2 Kerswell Cottages
Exminster, Exeter, Devon EX6 8AY, UK

Findhorn Flower Essences
The Wellspring, 31 The Park,
Findhorn Bay, Forres IV36 0TY, UK
Tel: 01309 690129
Fax: 01309 691300

Himalayan Flower Essences
Dr A Shah
15E Jaybharat Society
3rd Road, Khar
Bombay 400-052
INDIA

South African Flower & Gem Essences
PO Box F1
Constantia 7848
Cape
SOUTH AFRICA

Shell Essences
PO Box 984
Sutherland
NSW 2232
AUSTRALIA

Desert Alchemy
PO Box 44189
Tucson
AZ 85733
USA

Flower Essence Pharmacy
2007 NE 39th Avenue
Portland
OR 97212
USA

Fleurs de Vie
The Flower Essence Co.
Boite Postale 2
01170 Chevry
FRANCE

HOMOEOPATHIC SUPPLIERS,
COMPLEX HOMOEOPATHY AND VEGA
PRACTITIONERS

Noma Ltd
Unit 3
1-16 Hollybrook Road
Off Winchester Road
Upper Shirley
Southampton SO1 6RB

Chinese medicine
British Medical Acupuncture Society
Newton House
Newton Lane
Lower Whitley
Warrington
Cheshire WA4 4JA

Register of Chinese Herbal Medicine
c/o Midsummer Cottage Clinic
Nether Westcote
Kingham
Oxfordshire OX7 6SD

Western herbalism
National Institute of Medical Herbalists
34 Cambridge Road
London SW11

Homoeopathy
British Homoeopathic Association
27a Devonshire Street
London WC1N 1RJ

Ainsworths Homoeopathic Pharmacy
38 New Cavendish Street
London W1M 7LH

Weleda (UK) Ltd
Heanor Road
Ilkeston
Derbyshire DE7 8DR

Nutritional therapy
The Society for the Promotion of Nutritional
Therapy
PO Box 47
Heathfield
East Sussex TN21 8ZX
(*Send £1 and sae*)

KINESIOLOGY

Health Kinesiology (UK & Europe)
Sea View House
Long Rock
Penzance
Cornwall TR20 8JP
Tel: 001736 719030

Health Kinesiology (USA/Canada)
Birdsall House
RR3 Hastings
Ontario
CANADA

COUNSELLING

British Association for Counselling
37a Sheep Street
Rugby
Warks CV21 3BX

CRISIS HELP

The Samaritans 0345 909090 (day or night)

OTHER ADDRESSES

National Osteoporosis Society
PO Box 10
Radstock
Bath
Avon BA3 3YB

Endometriosis Society
245a Coldharbour Lane
London SW9 8RR

Further Reading

FLOWER ESSENCES

Findhorn Flower Essences, Marion Leigh. Findhorn Press, Scotland, 1997.

Amazonian Gem & Orchid Essences, Andreas Korte, Antje & Helmut Hoffman. Findhorn Press, Scotland, 1997.

Australian Bush Flower Essences, Ian White. Findhorn Press, Scotland, 1993.

Alaskan Flower, Gem and Environmental Essences, Steve Johnson. Findhorn Press, Scotland, 1998.

Encyclopaedia of Flower Essences, Clare Harvey etc. Thorsons, London, 1995.

COMPLEMENTARY THERAPIES

Medical Marriage, Dr Cornelia Featherstone & Lori Forsyth. Findhorn Press, Scotland, 1997.

NATURAL HORMONES

DHEA: Unlocking the Secrets to the Fountain of Youth, Beth M Ley. BL Publications, Aliso Viejo, 1996.

Preventing and Reversing Osteoporosis, A Gaby. Prima Publishing, 1994.

Natural Progesterone, Dr JR Lee. BLL Publishing, California, 1993.

What Your Doctor May Not Tell You About the Menopause, Dr J Lee. (BCM Box 4315, London WC1N 3XX.)

CHINESE MEDICINE

Second Spring, H Lee Wolfe. Blue Poppy Press, Boulder, CO, 1990.

The Journal of Chinese Medicine (22 Cromwell Road, Hove, Sussex BN3 3EC)

YOGA

Clear Mind Open Heart Yoga (cards), Celia Hawe. Findhorn Press, Scotland, 1998.

HEALING & PSYCHOLOGY

Hands-On Spiritual Healing, Michael Bradford. Findhorn Press, Scotland, 1994. Video tape also available.

Healing the Cause: A Path of Forgiveness, Michael Dawson. Findhorn Press, Scotland, 1994.

Spirit Child: Healing the Wound of Abortion, Isabella Kirton. Findhorn Press, Scotland, 1998.

MENOPAUSE

Menopause Matters, Judy Hall & Robert Jacobs. Element Books, Shaftesbury, 1994.

Passage to Power, Leslie Kenton. Vermillion, London, 1996.

Red Moon: Understanding and Using the Gifts of the Menstrual Cycle, M Gray. Element Books, Shaftesbury, 1994.

Women of the Fourteenth Moon, Taylor and Coverdale Sumai (eds). The Crossing Press, Freedom, CA, 1991.

MAGAZINES

What Doctors Don't Tell You (4 Wallace Road, London N1 2PG, UK)

Proof (4 Wallace Road, London N1 2PG, UK)

Positive Health (51 Queens Square, Bristol BS1 4LJ, UK)

GODDESSES

Larousse Encyclopaedia of Mythology, Hamlyn, New York, 1972.

Sophia Goddess of Wisdom, Caitlin Matthews. Mandala, London, 1991.

Descent to the Goddess, Sylvia Brinton Perera. Inner City Books, Toronto, 1981.

The Ancient British Goddess, Kathy Jones. Ariadne Publications, 56 Whiting Road, Glastonbury, Somerset BA6 8HR.

Kali: the Feminine Force, Ajit Mookerjee. Thames & Hudson, London, 1988.

Mysteries of the Dark Moon, Demetra George. HarperSanFrancisco, 1992.

Goddesses in Everywoman, Jean Shinoda Bolen MD. HarperCollins, San Francisco, 1985.

The Crone, Barbara G Walker. HarperCollins, San Francisco, 1985.

The Myth of the Goddess, Anne Baring & Jules Cashford. Arkana, London, 1993.

Index

Y

Z

MEDICAL MARRIAGE

The New Partnership between Orthodox and Complementary Medicine

✳ A model for health care in the 21st century
✳ Comprehensive information on 63 complementary therapies
✳ Thought provoking essays to catalyse change

by Dr Cornelia Featherstone and Lori Forsyth

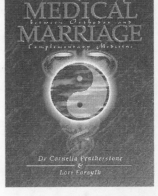

Written, compiled and edited by a medical doctor and a complementary practitioner, this book is an excellent example of co-operation. It epitomises the synergy which occurs when the two paradigms – the reductionist and the holistic – meet in mutual respect and open-mindedness: common ground is found and integrated health care becomes reality.

Patients are leading the way, as they are already making use of both complementary and orthodox medicine to increase their health care options. It is time for health care professionals in both fields to acknowledge each other's contributions and offer patients the quality of care which is only achievable through united and concerted action.

This book is essential reading for everyone interested in the field of health care. Doctors, nurses and complementary practitioners will find a wealth of information enabling them to work in multidisciplinary co-operation. Patients and conscious consumers will gain insight into the possibilities of integrated health care, allowing them to make educated choices about their own care.

Paperback 640 pages • ISBN 1 899171 16 9 • £19.95 • US$29.95 • CAN$39.95
Available from all good bookshops, or direct from
Findhorn Press for £19.95 including p&p

This is a warm, wonderful, thorough and above all honest exploration of a new medical dimension which is emerging out of mutually respectful teamwork between orthodox and complementary health care professionals... The messages which this book offers should be read – and above all applied – by every health care professional.
— **Leon Chaitow** ND DO
Consultant osteopath and naturopath
Marylebone Health Centre (NHS), London

...it is important that patients do take responsibility for their own health and furthermore it is important that doctors adopt a more co-operative and less pedagogic attitude to their patients and health care in general... so much of the book is excellent common sense, clearly written and a superb blueprint for the future.
— **Dr G T Lewith** MA DM MRCP MRCGP
Honorary Visiting Clinical Senior Lecturer
Southampton University

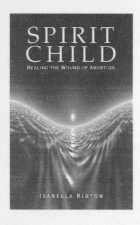

SPIRIT CHILD
HEALING THE WOUND OF ABORTION
Isabella M. Kirton

This is both a personal story and a self-help book for anyone who has aborted or miscarried an unborn child. Isabella already had three children and her decision to abort her fourth child was to have long-term repercussions, changing her life on all levels. Nine months from the conception of her child Isabella had a powerful phantom birth experience that impelled her into an altered reality. She decided not to turn to the simple solution of antidepressants, but tried truly to understand what was happening to her, finding that her intuitive and spiritual senses developed to help her. A powerful, yet sensitive book that offers support and understanding to women contemplating or having experienced abortion.

£6.95/us$11.95 Pbk 132 pages • ISBN 1 899171 12 6

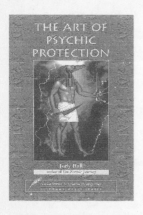

THE ART OF PSYCHIC PROTECTION
Judy Hall

A book of practical techniques and help for any individual or group seeking to expand their consciousness who need to protect themselves from psychic intrusion. For those who meditate, use guided imagery or self-hypnosis tapes, for therapists and healers, for those who find excessive tiredness a problem, the chances are that these people need to protect themselves with these tried and tested tools, some of which date back thousands of years whilst others belong to the 21st century. We protect ourselves in so many ways, we have tended to forget that psychic protection is a basic need.

£5.95 Pbk 144 pages • ISBN 1 899171 36 3

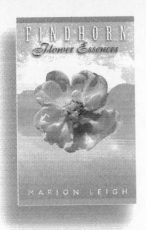

FINDHORN FLOWER ESSENCES

Marion Leigh

Marion explains the theory, pr eparation and practical applications of the flower essences. The book also includes a thor ough, indexed r epertoire of illnesses and their indicated tr eatments.

£9.95/us$16.95 Pbk 128 pages
ISBN 1 899171 96 7

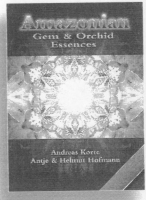

AMAZONIAN GEM & ORCHID ESSENCES

Andreas Korte, Antje & Helmut Hofmann

The vibratory qualities of Amazonian gems and orchids have been extracted for their therapeutic effects. This book describes each of the essences and its applications.

£9.95/us$16.95 Pbk 116 pages
(inc. 40 detachable colour cards)
ISBN 1 899171 91 6

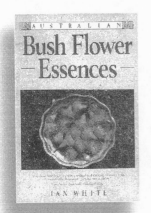

AUSTRALIAN BUSH FLOWER ESSENCES

Ian White

An informative yet personal pictur e of fifty bush flower essences and detailed infor mation about their preparation and use in all ar eas of healing. Fully illustrated. The Australian Bush Flower Essences themselves are available in the UK and many other countries.

£11.95/us$19.95 Pbk 210 pages (16 in colour)
ISBN 0 905249 84 4